SURGICAL FINALS

Passing the Clinical

D0726577

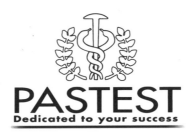

PASTEST
Dedicated to your success

To Marcia and Louis Kuperberg

SURGICAL FINALS

Passing the Clinical

Gina R Kuperberg BSc MBBS(Hons)
Registrar, The Maudsley Hospital, London.

John S P Lumley MS FRCS
Professor of Surgery, The University of London.
Honorary Consultant in Surgery,
St. Bartholomew's Hospital, London.
Council Member and Past Examiner in Anatomy for the
Royal College of Surgeons of England.

© 1996 PASTEST
Knutsford, Cheshire
WA16 8DX
Tel: 01565 752000

First published 1996. Reprinted 1996, 1998, 1999, 2000, 2001

ISBN 0 906896 38 X

A catalogue record for this book is available from the British Library,

The information contained within this book was obtained by the authors from reliable sources. However, while every effort has been made to ensure its accuracy, no responsibility for loss, damage or injury occasioned to any person acting or refraining from action as a result of information contained herein can be accepted by the publishers or authors.

PasTest Revision Books and Intensive Courses
PasTest has been established in the field of postgraduate medical education since 1972, providing revision books and intensive study courses for doctors preparing for their professional examinations. Books and courses are available for the following specialities:
MRCP Part 1 and 2 (General Medicine and Paediatrics), MRCOG, DRCOG, MRCGP, DCH, FRCA, MRCS, PLAB
For further details contact:
**PasTest, Freepost, Knutsford, Cheshire WA16 7BR
Tel: 01565 752000   Fax: 01565 650264**

Text prepared by Turner Associates, Caistor, Lincoln.
Printed and bound in Great Britain by Biddles
www.biddles.co.uk

CONTENTS

INTRODUCTION

By the end of clinical training, most students have accumulated enough knowledge to pass surgical finals. However, through poor organisation of the factual material, lack of confidence or examination stress, your performance may still be sub-optimal. This book is intended to reduce the chances of failure in the clinical part of the examination. It is not a comprehensive surgical text but provides relevant information for finals, particularly in the following areas:

- Useful tips for preparation of vivas and the long and short cases
- Relevant questions to include when taking a history in the long case
- Examination schemes designed to refine clinical skills in the short cases
- Examples of typical long and short cases, with lists of features, tables of differential diagnoses and common questions asked by examiners
- Popular viva questions which are ideal for self-assessment

The emphasis of this book is on a practical approach to clinical problems. The techniques described are applicable to the Final Examination and will keep your examiner happy. Additional checklists are provided to help you plan your revision. A concise, dogmatic and "no-frills" approach has been taken to allow rapid retrieval and packaging of information, the aim at all times being to minimise your examination difficulties.

GK
JSPL

ACKNOWLEDGEMENTS

We thank Dr Mark Gurnell, and the many medical students who have read the text, for their helpful comments and suggestions. Also Helen Turner for battling with the tables and endless proof corrections in earlier drafts of the book.
GK would like to thank Michael Jacobson for his support and computer expertise. Most of all, she acknowledges the unfailing encouragement of her parents, Marcia and Louis Kuperberg, who have consistently taught her to see a project through from idea to completion.

SYLLABUS CHECKLIST

As an aid to revision, use this syllabus as your own personal checklist. Page numbers are given in brackets after each case. You should aim to achieve at least two ticks per case before the date of the exam. If you have not actually seen a condition, look it up in an illustrated textbook.

Read

Seen/Taught on

Happy with

Pain, Swellings and Ulcers
1. Squamous cell papilloma / Skin tag (25)
2. Wart (26)
3. Seborrhoeic keratosis / Senile wart (26)
4. Pigmented naevus or malignant melanoma (26)
5. Dermatofibroma / Histiocytoma (27)
6. Pyogenic granuloma (27)
7. Keloid scar / Hypertrophic scar (27)
8. Keratoacanthoma / Molluscum sebaceum (28)
9. Keratin horn (28)
10. Sebaceous cyst (28)
11. Boil (28)
12. Hydradenitis suppurativa (29)
13. Strawberry naevus (29)
14. Port wine stain (30)
15. Lipoma (30)
16. Dermoid cyst (30)
17. Ganglion (30)
18. Venous ulcer (31)
19. Arterial ulcer (31)
20. Neuropathic ulcer (33)
21. Basal cell carcinoma (34)
22. Squamous cell carcinoma (34)

Neck Swellings and Thyroid Lumps
1. Goitre (46)
2. Thyroglossal cyst (49)
3. Cervical lymphadenopathy (51)
4. Parotid gland swelling (52)
5. Submandibular gland swelling (52)
6. Cervical rib (54)
7. Carotid body tumour (55)
8. Branchial cyst / sinus / fistula (55)

Read

Seen/Taught on

Happy with

COMPARISONS AND DIFFERENTIAL DIAGNOSES

Page numbers are given in brackets after each entry.

ABBREVIATIONS

The following abbreviations have been used throughout this book.

ASIS	anterior superior iliac spine
AV	arterio-venous
AXR	abdominal X-ray
CT	computerised tomography
CLL	chronic lymphocytic leukaemia
CXR	chest X-ray
DIP	distal interphalangeal
DVT	deep vein thrombosis
ECG	electrocardiogram
ENT	ear, nose and throat
FBC	full blood count
GIT	gastrointestinal tract
GP	general practitioner
HIV	human immunodeficiency virus
IP	interphalangeal
IVU	intravenous urogram
LFT	liver function tests
MCP	metacarpophalangeal
PIP	proximal interphalangeal
PR	per rectum
TB	tuberculosis
TFT	thyroid function tests
U&E	urea and electrolytes
UK	United Kingdom

1: THE CLINICAL: FORMAT AND PREPARATION

I. FORMAT

The clinical examination usually starts with a long case. Here, you are left alone with the patient to take a history and to perform a full examination. You are then shown into another room to present your findings. After this, the examiners will take you through a series of short cases.

The examiners

Examiners traditionally work in pairs. There is normally one 'internal' examiner (from your own teaching hospital) and one 'external' (invited from outside).

You will usually be told who your examiners are. It is worth knowing their special interests, even though their questions may not be confined to these areas. Talk to medical students who have been taught by your examiners to find out individual preferences in examination technique (for example, always kneeling down to examine the abdomen).

The patients

The range of conditions you will see in the examination is not necessarily representative of the conditions seen in general hospital care. Firstly, you will never be given a very ill patient, with, for example, an acute abdomen or an acutely ischaemic limb. Secondly, there are some rare conditions which crop up disproportionately in examinations: such patients usually have long-standing problems with good physical signs. Examples are AV malformations or carotid body tumours.

Patients are drawn from three sources:

a. <u>In-patients</u>

Most in-patients transferred to the examination will be awaiting operations such as hernia repairs or removal of breast lumps. However, there is an increasing tendency to include postoperative patients in the clinicals: after all, you will be expected to manage such patients as surgical house officers. A minority of patients will be those recovering from acute conditions, with good histories and/or physical signs that have not yet resolved.

b. Patients coming up from clinics

Patients with good physical signs who attend clinics in the few weeks before the clinicals are often asked to come up for the examination. Try and attend clinics in your hospital in the lead-up to finals. (For example, prior to surgical finals, one of the authors walked into the examination centre with a fellow candidate who pointed out two patients she recognised: "He has a sebaceous cyst on his forehead. She's got a left submandibular tumour". After revising these two conditions, she was given both patients as short cases!)

c. 'Professional' patients

These are patients with long-standing signs who are listed on a computer data base and have been called up numerous times in the past. Such patients are usually excellent historians and may even point out their physical signs.

II. PREPARATION

Early preparation

a. Don't fall into bad habits

Ask a doctor to watch you examine and listen to your presentations as early and as often as possible. Without this, it is very easy to acquire bad habits which are difficult to break.

b. Act as a chaperone

Fourth year medical students are often used as 'chaperones' in clinical examinations. Their role is to escort the candidates from room to room, ring the bells and ensure that the examination runs smoothly. If you are given this opportunity, take it. You will get an idea of the examination format and there will often be time to examine the patients yourselves afterwards. There can be no better preparation: some of the same patients may even come up the following year.

The revision period

a. Team up with a colleague

As the examination draws closer, pair up with a fellow student whose aims and standards are similar to your own and whose opinion you respect. By working in pairs, each of you can act as an examiner in turn, covering long and short cases and talking through topics that could arise in vivas. However, don't let anyone 'psyche you out': remember that each person works at his/her own pace and thinks the other knows more than him/herself. The relationship should be mutually beneficial.

b. Ask for senior help

During the revision period, don't hesitate to ask for extra teaching from senior staff: they've all been through finals themselves and are usually glad to help. Don't be put off by the tendency to teach by humiliation and don't worry if you are given different information or conflicting approaches: just extract what you consider the best information from each teacher.

Bleep the house officer and ask for lists of patients to see as long and short cases. Ask when patients are to be admitted. Also find out when day surgery lists take place: here you will find many swellings, ulcers, varicose veins and hernias to examine.

c. Revise efficiently

This book gives plenty of lists of clinical features and provides tables of differential diagnoses. Modify these to make your own lists: you will remember best what you compile yourself. A card system may be a useful revision aid at this stage.

Try not to work late into the night, relax before you go to bed, avoid excess coffee and keep up physical exercise. You will retain much more if you are alert during the revision period than if you are exhausted. Remember that hypnotics and anxiolytics may dull your mind on the day of the examination: take them only under medical supervision.

2: THE LONG CASE

This is usually the least stressful part of the clinical examination. However, don't underestimate it. It is surprising how many candidates present the long case in an incomplete and disorganised fashion.

Allocating your time

Be sure you know well in advance how much time you will be given for the long case. This varies from school to school. Normally, twenty minutes is the minimum. This provides very little time for complex peripheral vascular or GIT problems. If it looks as if the history will take longer than half the allotted time, start examining after you have taken the details of presenting complaint and past medical history. The remainder of the history can be taken at convenient points during the examination. It is essential that you practise this.

Rapport with the patient

It is important to establish a good rapport with your patient. Be friendly and polite. Make sure the patient is comfortable at all times. Do not ask the diagnosis immediately. On the other hand, if you gain the patient's sympathy, he/she may point you in the right direction and may even show you physical signs.

The history

Go through your usual scheme which should by now be familiar. Start with name, age, occupation and marital status. This is followed by seven headings:

(i) *Presenting complaint*
Ask about the main problem(s). List these together with a time scale, eg

- Abdominal pain: 3 weeks
- Nausea: 4 days

(ii) *History of presenting complaint*
Always include the systemic enquiry of the system relevant to the presenting complaint. Also ask the other appropriate questions (revised in sections of this book).

(iii) *Past medical and surgical history*
When asking about previous operations, remember to ask if there were any problems with the anaesthetic.

(iv) *Drug history and allergies*

(v) *Family history*
Again, include questions about anaesthetic reactions.

(vi) *Social history*
A good social history will make you stand out from other candidates. Don't just ask about alcohol and smoking. It is important that you know how well the patient will manage at home during the postoperative period. Therefore ask about family, neighbours, carers, GP home visits, district nurses, home help, meals on wheels and financial problems.

Your social history should be relevant to the patient's problem. For example, if you have a patient with a stoma, enquire into the details of stoma care. If you have a patient with an orthopaedic problem or amputation, ask about physiotherapy, occupational therapy, aids and appliances.

(vii) *Systemic enquiry*

The examination
Start your examination by forming a general impression of the patient. Look for **JACCOL** (**J**aundice, **A**naemia, **C**yanosis, **C**lubbing, **O**edema, **L**ymphadenopathy). In your systems approach, pay particular attention to the system relevant to the presenting complaint. However, aim to be thorough: *always* take the *pulse* and *blood pressure*. Remember to test the urine. A dipstick should be provided.

Thinking time
You will usually have a few minutes between examining the patient and presenting your findings. During this time, reorganise any misplaced information and summarise the case in writing. You might also predict your examiners' questions so that you are one step ahead. The sections on 'typical cases' in this book will help you to do this.

Presenting your findings

The examiners will usually tell you what they want. Normally, they will ask you to tell them about the patient you have just seen. They may add a rider such as "stick to the important features". Don't get flustered if they start with "What's the diagnosis?".

If your patient was a poor historian, start by commenting on this fact: this is an important sign in itself and allowances *will* be made. However, it is no excuse for a poor presentation.

Your presentation should be as concise, snappy and comprehensive as possible. Place your notes in front of you for reference but *talk*, don't read, to the examiners. Don't panic if your notes are taken away from you: the history and examination will be fresh in your mind and you will remember more than you think.

If the patient has more than one complaint, this should be brought out by *listing* the presenting complaints. Then explain, "I will describe each of these in turn".

You should not give long lists of negative findings: if the main problem is abdominal and you have found no other abnormality, it is quite permissible to state "other systems are normal".

The examiners may interrupt you in the middle of your presentation. They may be happy with the way you have started and want to go on to the next point, they may wish to discuss a problem in more depth, or they may simply be bored after listening to several well-delivered histories in a row.

You may be taken back to the patient to demonstrate an abnormal finding. This does not necessarily mean that there is any doubt about your findings: you may have elicited a sign previously missed!

3: THE SHORT CASES

The short cases are probably the most difficult part of the clinical examination. For the first time, you must examine a patient under the eagle eyes of two examiners.

The examiners will watch for three things:

A caring and competent approach

You should always introduce yourself. Fully expose the part of the body you wish to examine. Remember to compare both sides: if the examiner tells you to examine one leg, always expose the other as well. However, keep the patient 'decent'; for example, when exposing the legs, cover the groin. Before palpation, never forget to ask if there is any tenderness. The patient should be comfortable at all times. Thank the patient and cover him/her up before presenting your findings.

A good examination technique

Your examination of the short cases should be a smooth, thorough and slick performance. The only way to achieve this is to practise again and again so that the routine becomes second nature.

Note the following points:

- Do not take the examination schemes provided in this book as gospel. Modify them according to your own teaching and individual preference.

- Don't be such an automaton that you fail to listen to the instruction: if the examiner tells you to "palpate the abdomen", do not start with the hands.

- Passing the short cases is rather like passing a driving test: you must actually *show* your examiners that you are following the correct routine, for example, by standing at the end of the bed to observe the patient.

- Although you are not supposed to take a history during the short case, you *are* allowed certain questions. For example, before examining a lump you cannot see, ask the patient to point out its exact position.

- There are certain parts that you are not expected to include in the examination situation, such as a rectal examination. However, you *must* indicate to the examiners that you would normally examine these areas. Furthermore you should express a desire to examine other systems to seek underlying causes of local conditions. For example, tell the examiners that you would like to examine the abdomen for secondary causes of hernias or varicose veins.

- It is usually up to you whether you talk as you examine or present your findings at the end. Practise both ways: you may be requested specifically to "explain what you are doing" or you may be interrupted at any stage of the examination to "present your findings so far".

An ability to elicit and draw conclusions from physical signs

You will not fail the examination if you do not pick up all the physical signs. However, you will be asked questions such as "What are the causes of X?" and "What is the differential diagnosis?". Aim to be one step ahead of your examiners by pre-empting such questions.

Seek clues from the beginning: observe all the artefacts around the patient such as drips and catheters. Plastic gloves next to a patient with a submandibular swelling indicate that you are expected to palpate the gland bimanually. A glass of water next to a patient with a neck swelling suggests a goitre.

Never forget to look at the patient as a whole, even when you are asked to examine one small part: rheumatoid nodules on the elbow suggest the diagnosis before you have even looked at the hands.

4: THE VIVA

The viva itself lasts about twenty minutes, each examiner asking questions for ten minutes. You may particularly dread it as the field is vast and "they can ask you anything". However, examiners usually follow fairly standard approaches and, by practising and paying due attention to viva technique, it should not be too much of an ordeal.

You should be aware that any part of the clinical examination may turn into a 'mini-viva'. Indeed, the sections of this book entitled 'typical cases' deal specifically with the types of questions asked as part of long and short cases.

I. VIVA TECHNIQUE

Note the following points:

- Go in with a positive attitude.

- Although you will be nervous, try not to show it: aim to give an impression of calm confidence.

- Try to hold the attention of your examiners: speak audibly and clearly. Keep eye contact with at least one of them.

- When asked a question, consider for a moment before rushing into an answer. However, do not hesitate too long as this makes you appear uncertain.

- If you do not understand a question, admit it, put it behind you and be ready for the next question.

- Once you get onto a topic you know, keep talking as long as you have positive factual knowledge to offer. Drop your voice slightly on the final sentence so the examiners know you have completed your statement: try not to peter out.

- Be confident in your knowledge: avoid words such as "possible" and "I think". If an examiner says "are you sure?", this does not necessarily mean that you are wrong. If, however, an examiner tells you that you are wrong, accept it, even if you are certain you are right. This is not the time for argument or confrontation.

● Don't dig yourself a hole by mentioning a very rare condition or something about which you know little or nothing. The examiner could very well ask you to elaborate ("Oh yes, tell me more about that").

● Don't worry if some humour arises and you are excluded: examiners are pleased to have some light relief during a heavy day's examining. However, do not go out of your way to be funny as this can fall very flat.

● At the end, do not rush off as soon as the bell rings: the examiner decides the finishing point, not you. When the end is signalled, smile and thank the examiners, regardless of your feelings. Leave quietly at a normal pace. Try not to trip, knock over the chair or slam the door!

II. ORGANISATION OF INFORMATION

Always show the examiners that you can *classify* information.

A disease

You may be asked to talk about a particular disease. Use a pathology sieve to structure your answer. One aide-memoir is "Dressed In a Surgeon's Gown A Physician Might Make Progress": Definition, Incidence, Sex, Geography, Aetiology, Pathogenesis, Macroscopic pathology, Microscopic pathology, Prognosis. This can be slightly modified to form a clinical sieve "... a physician Should Succeed In Treatment": Symptoms, Signs, Investigations, Treatment.

Aetiology

Examiners often ask the causes of a condition. Remember to mention common causes before rarer ones. If you have not memorised a list for that condition, again refer to a sieve. You may find the following mnemonic useful: **CIMETIDINE**: Congenital, Infective/Inflammatory, Metabolic, Endocrine, Traumatic, Iatrogenic, Degenerative, Idiopathic, Neoplastic, Everything else!

Management

The question "How would you manage a patient with this condition?" comes up again and again. The term management is sometimes used loosely to be synonymous with treatment. However, management refers to history, examination, special investigations *and* treatment. You should *always* begin by saying "I would take a thorough history and perform a full examination". Go on to describe the special investigations you would request and only then describe the treatment. If asked about the management of trauma or shock, never forget to say: "This is an emergency. I would first check the airway, the breathing and the circulation".

Special investigations

When asked about special investigations, start with simple investigations such as urinalysis and blood tests: haematological (FBC, clotting studies, group and save) and biochemical (U&E, LFTs, TFTs, amylase). Then go on to describe relevant imaging investigations (CXR, ultrasound and dopplers, angiography, barium studies and CT scans) and biopsies (cytology and histology). Remember that all older patients being considered for surgery should have a CXR and ECG.

Treatment

If asked about the treatment of any disease, always divide your answer into conservative, medical, and surgical. Under conservative treatment, consider the contributions from all other providers such as nurses, physiotherapists, occupational therapists and social services. Under medical treatment, consider drugs, chemotherapy and radiotherapy.

III. TOPICS COVERED IN VIVAS

Objects used as talking points

Examiners will often have an array of objects in front of them which serve as useful talking points.

a. Results of investigations

Familiarise yourself with AXRs, barium studies, IVUs and angiograms. Examiners like to know if you have actually seen these investigations and may ask you to describe the procedures. You should also know normal haematological and biochemical values.

b. Pathology specimens

If handed a pathology pot, start by noting the organ. Then describe the abnormalities and make a diagnosis. Look all around the specimen: a discouraging amorphous mass on one view may be easily recognised by the presence of a nipple or an appendix on the other side. You may then be asked about the condition and how the patient presented.

c. Other objects

You are expected to recognise a variety of instruments and tubing. These include an endotracheal tube, a laryngoscope, a Guedel airway, a laryngeal mask, a chest drain, a tracheostomy tube, a Sengstaken-Blakemore tube, a T-tube, a proctoscope and a sigmoidoscope. You may be asked to describe a practical procedure such as how to catheterize or how to put down an endotracheal tube.

Other popular viva topics

Popular viva questions are listed at the end of each chapter in this book. You should be particularly aware of the following topics:

a. Emergencies

You *must* know about the management of the common surgical emergencies such as the acute abdomen and acute upper and lower GI bleeding. These are 'pass/fail' questions.

b. Anatomy and embryology

You are not expected to know much anatomy, embryology or details of operations. However, there are certain topics which are particularly popular with examiners. These include the anatomy of the inguinal and femoral canals, tracheostomy sites and the embryology of thyroglossal and branchial cysts.

c. General surgical care

It is essential that you know about fluid balance, postoperative complications and complications of fractures.

d. Topical questions

Keep an eye out for topical issues raised in the media and try to read the leaders of the Lancet or British Medical Journal.

5: THE DAY OF THE EXAMINATION

The examination week is very intensive. Each day covers long and short cases plus one or more vivas. It therefore deserves forethought and preparation, particularly on what you intend to take with you, what you will wear and how you will make your way to the examination.

Take appropriate equipment

Work out in advance exactly what you intend to carry. Know what equipment is in which pocket. Bring the following items:

- Watch with a second hand
- Stethoscope
- Short ruler
- Tape measure
- Pen torch (plus extra batteries)
- Opaque tube, eg an empty Smartie tube (for transillumination)
- Wooden spatulae (for looking in the mouth)
- Tourniquet (for examining varicose veins)

Neurological examination requires additional items which you can bring yourself. However, they will usually be provided.

- Cotton wool
- Sterile, sheathed disposable needles
- Tuning fork
- Tendon hammer
- Orange sticks (for eliciting plantar responses)
- Red and white-headed hat pins (each > 5mm diameter)
- Pocket-sized reading chart
- Ophthalmoscope

Dress conventionally

Avoid appearing at all unconventional. Men should wear a plain dark suit, tie and white shirt. Women should wear a smart dress or suit. Hair should be tidy: men should have a recent haircut and women with long hair should tie it back. Make sure your nails are clean and your shoes polished.

Arrive on time

It is essential that you arrive on time and in a composed state. You can be sure that there will be examiners and patients waiting for you, regardless of traffic delays or train strikes. Excuses wear thin on such occasions. If you are not familiar with the venue, a preliminary visit may be worthwhile in order to time your journey.

Aim to be at the examination at least thirty minutes before the listed starting time. This will ensure you are able to find the toilets, check your dress and equipment and fill in any necessary forms. It is a good idea, whilst waiting outside the examination room, to write down the various headings of your history and examination on the blank paper provided. Not only does this ensure you do not forget a heading in the heat of the situation, but it limits the space (and hence time) that you spend on any one area.

6: PAIN, SWELLINGS AND ULCERS

THE HISTORY

Pain, swellings and ulcers are presenting features of many diseases. Always ask the same questions:

Pain
— Where is the pain? (Ask the patient to point to the area where the pain is felt maximally.)
— Have you ever had a pain like this before?
— When did you first notice the pain this time?
— Did the pain begin suddenly or gradually?
— Has the pain become worse since it started?
— Can you describe the pain? (*?colicky ?burning ?aching*)
— How severe is the pain? Does it keep you awake at night?
— Does the pain go anywhere else?
— Is there anything that makes the pain better?
— Is there anything that makes the pain worse?
— What do you think caused the pain?

A mnemonic may help you remember the important features: **S**ite, **R**adiation, **S**everity, **N**ature, **O**nset, **P**eriodicity, **D**uration, **R**elieved by, **A**ccentuated by, **T**iming, (eg **S**tate **R**egistrered **S**taff **N**urse; **O**ut **P**atients **D**epartment; **RAT**).

A swelling or an ulcer
— When did you first notice it?
— How did you notice it?
— Has it changed since you first noticed it?
— Has it ever completely disappeared since you noticed it?
— How does it bother you? (What are the main symptoms: is it painful or tender?)
— Do you have (or have you ever had) any other lumps or ulcers?
— What do you think caused it?

THE EXAMINATION

Even if the diagnosis seems obvious, always go through the same routine when examining a swelling or an ulcer. It is probably easier to talk as you go rather than to present your findings at the end.

"Examine this patient's swelling"

ACTION	NOTE
– Introduce yourself	
– Ask permission to examine the patient	
– Expose the lump completely	
LOOK	
– Inspect the lump	*?shape* *?colour*
– Measure: • distance from the nearest bony prominence	*?position*
• dimensions	*?size*
FEEL	
– Ask if the lump is tender/painful	Note if any part is sensitive on subsequent palpation
a. <u>Temperature</u>	
– Run the backs of your fingers over the surface and surrounding area	*?warm*

b. Surface

– Feel with the pulps of your fingers

?smooth
?bosselated
?rough

c. Edge

– Feel with your finger and thumb

?clearly/poorly defined

d. Consistency

?stony-hard
?rubbery-hard
?spongy
?soft

e. Surrounding area

?indurated

PRESS

a. Pulsatility

– Rest a finger of each hand on opposite sides of the lump for a few seconds
Watch your fingers

?expansile pulsation (fingers pushed apart)
?transmitted pulsation (fingers pushed in same direction)

b. Compressibility/ Reducibility

– Press the lump firmly and then release the pressure

?compressible (lump disappears on pressure and reappears on release)
?reducible (lump reappears only on application of another force, eg coughing, gravity)

c. Percussion

– Percuss over lump

?*dull*
?*resonant*

d. Fluctuation/Fluid Thrill

– Place two fingers of one
hand at opposite ends of
the lump
Press the middle of the
lump with the index
finger of your other
hand

Use this test for a *small*
lump

?*fluctuant*
(two fingers move apart when
middle area pressed)

– Repeat in a perpendicular
plane

– Ask patient to place the
edge of his/her hand in
the middle of the
swelling
Flick on one side and
feel on other side for a
percussion wave

Use this test for a *large*
swelling

?*fluid thrill*

MOVE

– Try to move the skin
over the lump

?*fixation to skin*
(skin cannot be moved over
lump)

– Try to move the lump in
two planes at right
angles to each other

?*mobility*

– Ask patient to tense the
underlying muscle
Reassess mobility

?*attachment to underlying
muscle* (movement *reduced* when
underlying muscle tensed)

LISTEN

– Auscultate over the lump

?bruit
?bowel sounds

TRANSILLUMINATE

– Press a pen torch and an
opaque tube (eg a
Smartie tube) on
opposite sides of the
lump
Look down the opaque
tube

?transilluminable
(transillumination can only
be accurately assessed by
looking down the opaque tube)

EXAMINE SURROUNDING TISSUES

– Examine regional lymph
nodes:
(limbs/trunk: axillary
nodes
head/neck: cervical
nodes)

?local lymphadenopathy

– Test sensation in the
surrounding area

?local neurological deficit

– Test the power of related
muscles

"Examine this patient's ulcer"

<u>ACTION</u>	<u>NOTE</u>	
LOOK		
– Measure:		
• distance from the nearest bony prominence		*?position*
• dimensions		*?size*
		?shape
– Inspect the base	colour:	*?red/granulation tissue*
	penetration:	*?tendon*
		?bone
	discharge:	*?blood*
		?pus
– Inspect the edge	edge:	*?flat sloping*:

?punched out:

?undermined:

?raised:

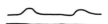

?raised and everted:

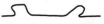

| – Measure the depth in mm | *?depth* | |

FEEL

– Ask if the surrounding
area is tender

– Feel with the backs of
your fingers

?warm

**EXAMINE SURROUNDING
TISSUES**

– Examine the regional
lymph nodes

?local lymphadenopathy

– Test sensation in the
surrounding area

?local neurological deficit

– Test the power of related
muscles

TYPICAL CASES

I. LUMPS AND SWELLINGS

Neck, breast, abdomen and knee swellings are covered on pages 46-56, 63-65, 83-87, and 154-156. This section revises skin lumps, giving examples of common short cases.

Lesions derived from the epidermis

Case 1: *Squamous cell papilloma / Skin tag*
This is a pedunculated overgrowth of skin. It is soft, the colour of normal skin and may occur at any site.

Case 2:   Wart

Warts are grey/brown filiform lesions, usually seen on the back of the hand. The *surface* is rough and the *consistency*, hard.

Case 3:   Seborrhoeic keratosis / Senile wart

These are flattened, well-defined plaques, usually found on the back. They may be multiple and are usually pigmented. The patient will probably be elderly. They are easily recognised because of their *greasy, rough surface* and because they are *easy to pick off* (although you should not try to do this if you are uncertain of the diagnosis).

Case 4:   Pigmented naevus or malignant melanoma

Benign naevi may occur anywhere. They may be flat, raised, hairy or non-hairy. The surface may be rough or smooth.

You should know the characteristics that suggest malignancy:

- Increase in size
- Ulceration
- Change in colour
- Irritation
- Bleeding
- Halo of pigmentation
- Satellite nodules
- Enlarged local lymph nodes
- Evidence of distant spread

Note: squamous cell and basal cell carcinomas may also present as epidermal nodules. They usually ulcerate and are considered in section II, page 34.

Lesions derived from the dermis

Case 5: *Dermatofibroma / Histiocytoma*

This is a firm nodule, usually seen on the lower leg. It is part of the skin and fully mobile.

Case 6: *Pyogenic granuloma*

This is a bright-red or blood-encrusted nodule. It feels fleshy and is slightly compressible. It bleeds easily.

If you are not sure of the diagnosis, ask the patient how quickly it appeared (it arises within days) and whether he/she remembers a preceding penetrating injury.

Note: unlike its name implies, it is *not* granulomatous *or* pyogenic. It is actually an acquired haemangioma.

Case 7: *Keloid scar*

Keloid is an overgrowth of fibrous tissue within a scar. Suspect this in a black patient who has had a recent operation.

You may be asked about the differences between a *keloid* and a *hypertrophic* scar:

	HYPERTROPHIC SCAR	**KELOID SCAR**
Overall Incidence	More common	Less common
Association with race?	No	Yes: more common in Afro-Caribbean people
Extent of overgrowth	Confined to scar tissue	Extends into surrounding tissue
Resolves spontaneously?	Yes: within a few months	No
Recurs after surgery?	No	Yes

Lesions derived from skin appendages

Case 8:   Keratoacanthoma / Molluscum sebaceum

A keratoacanthoma is a benign overgrowth of a sebaceous gland.
It appears within 3-4 weeks. It resembles a volcano, consisting of a conical lump of normal skin colour with a *central crater* containing keratin. It usually regresses spontaneously but may take 6-9 months.

Case 9:   Keratin horn

This is a dry, hard spike, derived from sebaceous secretions.
Unlike a keratoacanthoma, it does *not* regress.

Case 10: Sebaceous cyst

This is an extremely common short case. It is usually found in hairy areas (the scalp, neck, face and scrotum).
The size varies but the lump is usually hemispherical with a well-defined edge. Although it lies subcutaneously, it *is* attached to skin by the sebaceous duct.
The *consistency* is hard although there is some fluctuation. It is *not* usually transilluminable.
Always look for a punctum: only 50% will possess one but it is pathognomonic if you find it.
If the cyst is painful and red, this does not necessarily indicate infection: following trauma, the secretions may cause a foreign body inflammatory response in the surrounding tissues. Bacteria, however, cannot usually be cultured.
If you are asked about its origin, remember that the term 'sebaceous' cyst is a misnomer. It is *not* derived from the sebaceous gland, but from the outer sheath of the hair follicle. The cyst contents, although thick and waxy, are dead epithelial elements rather than sebaceous secretions.

Case 11: Boil

A boil or furuncle is an infection originating in a hair follicle. It begins as a hard, red tender lesion. It later discharges spontaneously.
If you are allowed to ask the patient a few questions, ask about diabetes, steroid therapy and other predisposing immunodeficiencies.

You may be asked to describe the differences between a furuncle and a carbuncle:

	FURNUNCLE	**CARBUNCLE**
Site	Skin	Subcutaneous tissue
Number of abscesses seen	One	Several
Appearance	Discrete lesion	Generalised necrotic area

Case 12: *Hydradenitis suppurativa*

A red, tender swelling is not necessarily a boil: if the patient has *multiple* such lesions in the *axillae* or *groin*, suspect hydradenitis suppurativa — infection of sweat glands.

Lesions derived from vascular structures

The term 'haemangioma' encompasses many lesions, including Campbell de Morgan spots and spider naevi.

You should also be able to recognise the two common paediatric haemangiomata:

Case 13: *Strawberry naevus*

This is a bright-red, strawberry-like lesion. It is small at birth but increases in size and may be disfiguring. It should be left alone, as it spontaneously regresses by the age of about 4-5. Remember the important exception to this rule is when it obscures a visual field.

Case 14: *Port wine stain*

As its name implies, this is a flat purple/red lesion with an irregular border. It is present at birth and does not increase or decrease in size thereafter.

Lesions not attached to skin

Case 15: *Lipoma*

This is a benign tumour of adipocytes. Its size varies. The *shape* is hemispherical and the *edge* is well-defined. The *consistency* is soft and the *surface*, bosselated.

Note: only *large* lipomas are fluctuant and transilluminable.

Lipomas are usually freely mobile although they may occasionally lie beneath the deep fascia.

Case 16: *Dermoid cyst*

Dermoid cysts are hard and spherical. Although derived from epithelial elements within the dermis, they lie subcutaneously.

In an adult, you should suspect an *implantation* dermoid, usually found on the fingers. Ask about a preceding injury.

In a child, suspect a *congenital* dermoid. This occurs at the sites of fusion of the facial processes, eg the outer angle of the eye.

Case 17: *Ganglion*

The patient will have a smooth, hemispherical swelling near a joint or tendon. The most common sites are at the wrist, on the dorsum of the forearm and around the ankle. The *surface* is smooth and the *consistency*, firm. It is slightly fluctuant and weakly transilluminable.

Remember to palpate the ganglion in all positions of the underlying joint: its mobility depends on whether it is derived from, and thus attached to, deep structures.

Note that the origin is controversial. Some view it as a pocket of synovium, communicating with the associated joint. Others see it as a myxomatous degeneration of fibrous tissue, derived from the tendon sheath.

II. ULCERS

You should know the definition of an ulcer: a defect in an epithelial surface. You may be asked the causes:

TYPE	CAUSE	UNDERLYING DISEASE
Venous (page 127) (75% of leg ulcers)	(i) *Superficial venous insufficiency* (ii) *Deep venous insufficiency*	• Varicose veins • Previous DVT
Arterial (page 118)	(i) *Large vessel disease (ischaemic)*	• Atheroma • Beurger's disease
	(ii) *Small vessel disease (vasculitis)*	• Rheumatoid arthritis • Polyarteritis nodosa
Traumatic	(i) *Neuropathic/trophic*	• Alcohol • Diabetes mellitus • Tabes dorsalis • Syringomyelia
	(ii) *Others*	• Bedsores • Self-inflicted injury
Infective	*Often associated with malnutrition*	• Pyogenic organisms • Tertiary syphilis • Mycobacterium ulcerans
Neoplastic	(i) *Primary neoplasm*	• Squamous cell carcinoma • Basal cell carcinoma • Malignant melanoma
	(ii) *Secondary neoplasm*	

Case 18: *Ulcer with a sloping edge*

A sloping edge is characteristic of a *healing* ulcer, ie a *traumatic* (although not neuropathic) ulcer or a *venous* ulcer.

Venous ulcers are found in the 'gaiter area' (above the malleoli, particularly the *medial* malleolus). They are usually shallow and flat. The *base* is covered with pink granulation tissue mixed with white fibrous tissue.

Look for and describe associated signs of superficial or deep venous insufficiency (see page 128).

Case 19: *Ulcer with a 'punched-out' edge*

It is unlikely that you will see a gumma of tertiary syphilis which is the classic 'punched-out' ulcer. This usually occurs on the anterior aspect of the lower leg and is easily recognised by the yellow-coloured ('wash-leather') base.

Ischaemic and neuropathic ulcers are much more common short cases. They have many of the same characteristics:

- Over the tips and between toes
- Over pressure areas (heel, malleoli)
- Pale pink base (very *little* granulation tissue)
- Deeply penetrating
- Bone, ligaments and tendons seen in the base

Ischaemic ulcers are secondary to circulatory insufficiency (large or small vessel disease) whereas *neuropathic ulcers* are usually secondary to spinal cord disease or a peripheral neuropathy: repeated injury arises from loss of pain. Remember that diabetes mellitus has a *mixed* pathogenesis (see page 118).

If you are asked to distinguish between the two, use the following scheme:

	ISCHAEMIC ULCER	**NEUROPATHIC ULCER**
Ask if the ulcer is painful	Painful	Painless
Look for associated black eschar	Present	Absent
Feel the temperature of the surrounding area	Cold	Warm
Test the sensation of the the surrounding area	Sensation intact	Sensation lost

Case 20: *Ulcer with a raised edge*

Ulcers with raised edges are neoplastic. The centre of the carcinoma becomes necrotic, but the periphery continues to grow and rises above the surface of the surrounding skin.

The main features distinguishing a basal cell carcinoma (rodent ulcer) from a squamous cell carcinoma are the *edge* and the *colour*:

	BASAL CELL CARCINOMA	SQUAMOUS CELL CARCINOMA
Edge	Raised , rolled	Raised and everted
Colour	Pearly, glistening, pink tinge (due to fine telangiectasia)	Red-brown (due to vascularity)

You should be able to list the predisposing factors for skin cancer:

- Age
- Sunlight (ultraviolet radiation)
- Ionizing radiation
- Chemical irritants (eg soot, dyes, tar)

Remember that malignant change (usually to squamous cell carcinoma) may also occur in long-standing benign ulcers (Marjolin's ulcers), in scars and in chronically discharging osteomyelitis sinuses.

POPULAR VIVA QUESTIONS

— Describe the features you would note in examining a lump/an ulcer. How would these features help in your differential diagnosis?

— What is the difference between a furuncle and a carbuncle?

— What are the differences between a keloid and hypertrophic scar?

— What are the features that would suggest malignancy in a pigmented naevus?

— Describe the differences in appearance between a basal cell carcinoma and a squamous cell carcinoma.

— What aetiological factors may predispose to squamous cell carcinoma?

7: NECK SWELLINGS AND THYROID LUMPS

THE HISTORY

If your patient complains of a swelling in the neck, ask the same questions as for any lump (page 19).

If you suspect lymphadenopathy, ask the following questions to determine *local* causes:
- Do you have any mouth ulcers or pain in your mouth?
- Do you have any pain or discharge from your nose or ears?
- Do you have a sore throat?
- Have you noticed any other lumps on your head or face?
- Do you have any difficulty swallowing?
- Do you have any difficulty breathing?

Your systemic enquiry will be important in determining *generalised* causes.

If you suspect a goitre, ask the following specific questions:

Local effects of the swelling
- Is the lump painful?
- Do you have any difficulty or pain when you swallow?
- Do you have any difficulty breathing?
- Have you noticed any change in your voice recently?

Eye problems associated with hyperthyroidism
- Do you have double vision?
- Do you get painful, red eyes?

Systemic enquiry to determine thyroid status

a. General symptoms:

- Have you noticed a change in your appearance?
- Are you intolerant of hot or cold temperatures?

b. Gastro-intestinal symptoms:

- Have you noticed a change in your appetite/weight/bowel habit?

c. Cardiorespiratory symptoms

 — Do you get palpitations/shortness of breath on exertion/ankle swelling/chest pain?

d. Neurological symptoms

 — Have you noticed any nervousness/irritability/insomnia/loss of concentration?

e. Gynaecological symptoms *(in females)*:

 — Have you noticed any change in your menstrual cycle?

THE EXAMINATION

A common instruction in the short case is to "examine this patient's neck" without being given any clue as to the pathology. Alternatively, you may be asked to "examine this patient's thyroid gland". In this case, proceed to the relevant section of the examination scheme below. Rarely, you may be pointed out a lump and asked to describe it (pages 20-23).

The presence of a glass of water near the patient is a good hint that there may be a goitre!

Always describe the position of neck swellings in terms of the triangles of the neck:

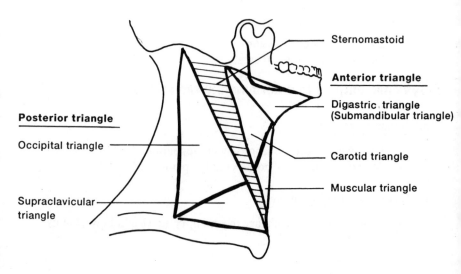

"Examine this patient's neck"

<u>ACTION</u>	<u>NOTE</u>
– Introduce yourself	
– Ask permission to examine the patient	
– Expose the neck, with the patient sitting up comfortably	
LOOK	
– Observe from in front and from either side	*?hyperaemia of skin* *?scars* *?distended neck veins* *?obvious goitre* (between thyroid cartilage and manubrium sterni)
– Ask patient to take a sip of water and to hold it in his/her mouth Then ask patient to swallow	*?goitre* (moves on swallowing)
– Ask patient to stick out tongue	*?thyroglossal cyst* (moves up when tongue stuck out)

NOW PROCEED AS FOLLOWS:

- *If obvious goitre*, continue examination of thyroid gland: **I** (page 40)

- *If no goitre*, examine for cervical lymphadenopathy: **II** (page 43)

- *If you feel an obvious lump*, proceed to **III** (page 44)

- *If you suspect enlargement of a salivary gland*, proceed to **IV** (page 45)

I. Examination of Thyroid Gland

ACTION	NOTE
LOOK (see above)	
FEEL	
– Stand behind patient	
– Ask if the swelling is tender	
– Feel with the flat of your fingers over the thyroid (thumbs posteriorly)	
– Tell patient to take another sip of water, hold it in his/her mouth and then to swallow	*?thyroid felt to move on swallowing*
– Palpate gently	*?tender*
	?diffusely-enlarged swelling
	?single nodule
	?multinodular goitre
	?texture
	?surface
	?approximate size
– Palpate the cervical lymph nodes	*?associated lymphadenopathy* (page 43)
– Whilst still standing behind patient, look over the top of his/her head	*?exophthalmos*
ASSESS POSITION	
– Stand in front of patient	
– Palpate the trachea in the suprasternal notch	*?trachea deviated*
– Percuss the thyroid	*?lower limit of retrosternal extension*
– Auscultate over the thyroid	*?bruit*

ASSESS THYROID FUNCTION

a. Observe overall

Look at patient's:
- face and skin ?*dry/shiny skin*
- build ?*thin/fat*
- dress ?*appropriate for temperature*
- behaviour ?*agitated/lethargic*

b. Examine the hands

– Look at:
- palms ?*palmar erythema*
- nails ?*thyroid acropachy*

– Feel:
- palms ?*sweaty*
- pulse ?*large volume*
  ?*atrial fibrillation*

– Ask patient to hold arms ?*fast postural tremor*
outstretched

c. Examine the eyes

– Look at:
- conjunctiva ?*chemosis/oedema/redness*
- relationship of
  eyelid to iris ?*lid retraction*

– Ask patient to follow your
finger up and down ?*lid lag*

– Test the eye movements:
Ask patient to follow a white
hat pin with eyes
Ask him/her to report any ?*ophthalmoplegia*
double vision

d. <u>Assess neurologically</u>

– Ask patient to rise from a
squatting position (or chair)
without using hands for support

?proximal myopathy
(a sensitive indicator of
hypo/hyperthyroidism)

– Test reflexes, observing the
relaxation phase:
- supinator
- biceps

?slow-relaxing reflexes
(suggests hypothyroidism)

II. Examination for cervical lymphadenopathy

ACTION	NOTE
– Stand behind patient – Examine lymph nodes *systematically:*	

First feel the horizontal ring:
    • submental
    • submandibular
    • preauricular
    • postauricular
    • occipital	

Then feel the vertical chain:
    • deep cervical
    • posterior triangle
    • supraclavicular
	?position of enlarged nodes

If you feel enlarged cervical lymph nodes,	
– Look in the mouth, ears and throat with pen-torch – Say you would request a full ENT examination – Look carefully at the face and all over the scalp	*?primary site of infection* *?primary malignancy*

– Examine:
    • epitrochlear nodes
    • inguinal nodes
    • axillary nodes
	?generalised lymphadenopathy

– Examine patient above the umbilicus	*?skin lumps* *?normal respiratory system* *?breast lumps*
– Examine the abdomen	*?splenomegaly ?hepatomegaly*

III. Examination of other neck lumps

<u>ACTION</u>	<u>NOTE</u>
– Assess as for any lump (pages 20-23)	*?neck triangle* *?shape* *?colour* *?size* *?temperature* *?surface* *?edge* *?consistency*
– Palpate lump as patient contracts the underlying muscle: eg *sternomastoid*: tell patient to push chin against your hand (away from the side of the lump) eg *trapezius*: tell patient to shrug his/her shoulders as you push down	*?fixation to underlying muscle*
– Examine for cervical lymphadenopathy (as above)	*?associated lymphadenopathy*

IV. Examination of a Salivary Gland

ACTION	NOTE
– Assess as for any lump (pages 20-23)	*?position* *?shape* *?colour* *?size* *?temperature* *?surface* *?edge* *?consistency*
– Look inside the mouth: observe submandibular papillae (on either side of the frenulum) and the parotid duct orifice (opposite the second upper molar tooth)	Duct orifice: *?inflamed* *?pus/exudate*
– Feel inside the mouth: bimanually palpate submandibular gland	A box of plastic gloves nearby suggests this is expected *?relation to tongue* *?relation to floor of mouth* *?tenderness*
– Feel along duct	*?stone*
– If you suspect enlargement of the parotid gland, test 7th nerve: "screw up your eyes; blow out your cheeks; whistle"	*?facial nerve palsy*

TYPICAL CASES

I. MIDLINE NECK SWELLINGS

You should memorise a list of midline neck swellings:

COMMON	• Thyroid swellings • Thyroglossal cyst
UNCOMMON	• Lymph nodes • Sublingual dermoid cyst • Plunging ranula • Pharyngeal pouch • Subhyoid bursa • Carcinoma of larynx/trachea/oesophagus

Case 1: *Goitre*

Revise the causes of a goitre:

a. <u>Physiological</u>

  • Puberty
  • Pregnancy

b. <u>Simple colloid goitre and multinodular goitre</u>

  Note: these have the same underlying pathogenesis and a *multifactorial aetiology:*

  • Goitregens
  • Dyshormogenesis
  • Iodine deficiency (epidemic, endemic)
  • Autoimmune

c. Autoimmune thyroid disease

> • Hashimoto's thyroiditis
> • Graves' disease

d. Other thyroiditides

> • de Quervain's (acute)
> • Riedel's (chronic fibrosing)

e. Tumours

(i) *Benign*
(ii) *Malignant*
> • Primary (carcinoma)
> • Secondary (lymphoma)

f. Other
> • Tuberculosis
> • Sarcoidosis

Note that if you feel a single nodule, you may be feeling the following:

• One nodule of a multinodular goitre
• An enlarged lobe (eg malignant infiltration; Hashimoto's thyroiditis)
• A true single nodule, ie a neoplasm. This may be *benign* (adenoma: functional or non-functional) or *malignant*.

You may be asked about the different kinds of primary thyroid cancers:

TYPE	NOTE
Papillary	Lump may be situated anterolaterally: otherwise known as 'lateral aberrant thyroid'; actually an involved lymph node
Follicular	Ask about bone pain (metastasizes via blood)
Medullary	Lump feels stony hard due to amyloid infiltration
Anaplastic	Usually middle-aged or elderly patients Not a discrete lump because of infiltration into surrounding tissues

Assess thyroid status independently: you are expected to know the common
causes of hyper and hypothyroidism:

	CAUSE	NOTE
Hyperthyroidism	Graves' disease	• Autoimmune • Younger patients • Goitre is diffusely enlarged with bruit
	Multinodular goitre	• Older patients
	Functioning adenoma	• Rare • Most are non-functioning
Hypothyroidism	Primary myxoedema	• Autoimmune • Older patients • No goitre
	Hashimoto's thyroiditis	• Autoimmune • Younger patients • Rubbery goitre • At an early stage, patient may be hyperthyroid

Case 2: *Thyroglossal cyst*

This is a spherical midline lump. It feels hard and the edge is clearly defined.
Ask the patient to stick out his/her tongue: the lump will move *up* due to its
attachment to the fibrous remnants of the thyroglossal tract.
Note its position: is it suprahyoid or infrahyoid?
You may find it difficult to fluctuate and to transilluminate.

II. LATERAL NECK SWELLINGS

Don't forget that an asymmetrical thyroid swelling may *appear* as a lateral neck swelling.

Otherwise, think of lateral swelling as derived from paired lateral structures. Don't forget that lymph nodes are by far the most common cause.

	ANTERIOR TRIANGLE	POSTERIOR TRIANGLE
Lymph nodes	• Lymph node • Cold abscess*	• Lymph node • Cold abscess*
Salivary glands	• Submandibular swelling • Parotid swelling	
Cystic structures	Branchial cyst	Cystic hygroma
Vascular structures	• Carotid body tumour • Carotid body aneurysm	Subclavian artery aneurysm
Other structures	Sternomastoid 'tumour' (ischaemic contracture)	Tumour of clavicle

* *Note*: a cold abscess arises from TB involvement of the nodes: the caseating nodes *point*, weakening the overlying tissue and then *burst*, causing a 'collar-stud' abscess.

Case 3: Cervical lymphadenopathy

You are likely to be asked the differential diagnosis:

	LOCALISED LYMPHADENOPATHY	GENERALISED LYMPHADENOPATHY
Infective	• Tonsillitis • Laryngitis • Infected skin lesion, eg sebaceous cyst • TB • Toxoplasmosis	(i) *Acute* • Infectious mononucleosis • Cytomegalovirus (ii) *Chronic* • TB • Brucellosis • Secondary syphilis • HIV
Neoplastic	Metastases from carcinoma of: • Head and neck • Breast • Chest • Abdomen	(i) *Lymphoma* • Hodgkin's • Non-Hodgkin's (ii) *Leukaemias* eg CLL
Other		• Amyloidosis • Sarcoidosis

Case 4: Salivary gland swelling

You may be given a patient with enlargement of the parotid or submandibular glands.

Be able to classify the causes of salivary gland enlargement:

a. Infection: (sialoadenitis)

    (i) *Acute*   • Viral
                    • Bacterial

    (ii) *Recurrent* • *Obstructive*: calculus, stricture
                      • *Non-obstructive*: children, menopausal females

    (iii) *Chronic* • Tuberculosis
                      • Actinomycosis

b. Autoimmune

                      • Sicca syndrome
                      • Sjogren's syndrome

c. Calculi (sialolithiasis)

d. Cysts

                      • Simple cysts (parotid)
                      • Mucous retention cysts

e. Infiltration

                      • Sarcoidosis

f. Systemic disease

                      • Alcoholic liver cirrhosis
                      • Diabetes mellitus
                      • Pancreatitis
                      • Acromegaly
                      • Malnutrition

g. Drugs

- Phenothiazines
- Phenylbutazone

h. Allergy

- Iodine

i. Malignancy

- Benign
- Intermediate
- Malignant

Remember:

- 80% of salivary *neoplastic* conditions occur in the *parotid* gland.
- Most *stones* occur in the *submandibular* gland.

The most likely cause of parotid enlargement is a benign mixed parotid tumour. Occasionally you will see Warthin's tumour. The following characteristics distinguish these two tumours:

	MIXED PAROTID TUMOUR	WARTHIN'S TUMOUR
Position	Just above and anterior to jaw angle	Slightly lower: lower border of mandible
Consistency	Rubbery-hard	Soft
Mobility	+	+ +
Fluctuant?	No	Yes

You may be asked how you would clinically assess the *malignancy* of a parotid tumour. The distinguishing features are:

- Short presentation
- Painful
- Hyperaemic and hot skin
- Hard consistency
- Fixed to skin and underlying muscle
- Irregular surface and indistinct edge
- Invasion of facial nerve

Case 5: *Cervical rib*

This rarely comes up in examinations.
The lump is only occasionally palpable, just above the clavicle. It may be pulsatile due to the elevated subclavian artery.

Look out for neurological and vascular features:

(i) *Neurological Features* (more common)
- Pain in C8 and T1 dermatomes
- Wasting and weakness of small muscles of the hand

(ii) *Vascular Features* (rarer)
- Raynaud's phenomenon
- Rest pain
- Trophic changes
- Gangrene

Case 6: *Carotid body tumour*

This is a rare condition but may come up in the examination as a short case. The tumour feels hard and is otherwise known as a 'potato tumour'. The position is shown below.

You may feel pulsation. This may result from the following sources:

- Internal carotid artery (transmitted)
- External carotid artery (running superficially)
- Tumour itself (intrinsic vascularity)

— Ask about blackouts, transient paralysis and paraesthesia.
— Check the other side: the tumour is often bilateral.

Case 7: *Branchial cyst / sinus / fistula*

Note that, although these are *developmental*, arising from remnants of the second pharyngeal pouch, they present in young adults.
The cyst has a distinct edge and a smooth surface. Depending on its contents, it may or may not transilluminate.

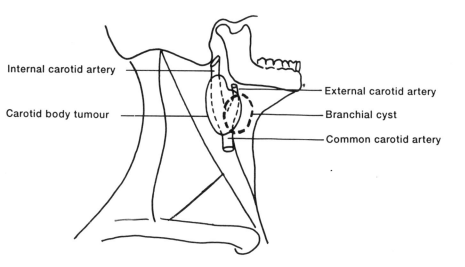

You may be shown a branchial sinus or fistula - a small dimple in the skin, at the junction of the middle and lower third of the anterior edge of sternomastoid.

— Ask the patient to swallow: this will make it more obvious.
— Ask about discharge.

Know the *definitions* of a sinus and a fistula:

Sinus: a blindly-ending track, leading away from an epithelial surface into surrounding tissue, lined by epithelial or granulation tissue.
(In this instance, there is no closing off of the second branchial cleft, although the upper end is obliterated.)

Fistula: an abnormal tract connecting two epithelial surfaces, lined by epithelial or granulation tissue.
(In this instance, the fistula connects skin to the oropharynx, just behind the tonsil.)

POPULAR VIVA QUESTIONS

— What are the causes of cervical lymphadenopathy?

— What are the possible causes of a lump in the anterior triangle of the neck?

— What are the causes of a thyroid swelling?

— What are the causes of hyper and hypothyroidism?

— What are the indications for the surgical management of hyperthyroidism?

— What precautions would you take in preparing a patient with hyperthyroidism for surgery?

— What are the complications of thyroidectomy?

— What kinds of thyroid malignancy do you know?

— What are the causes of stones in the salivary ducts? Where are they most likely to form?

— What is the most common tumour of the parotid gland? How should it be managed?

— What clinical features distinguish a benign from a malignant salivary tumour?

— What are the sites of the openings of the submandibular and parotid ducts into the mouth?

— What are the complications of surgery to the parotid gland?

8: THE BREAST

Your patient in either the long or short case may be a woman complaining of pain or a lump in her breast.

THE HISTORY

Bring out the following points when presenting under 'history of presenting complaint':

Breast lump
— When did you notice the lump? How did you notice it?
— Has the lump *changed* since you first noticed it? How?
— Is it painful?
— Have you had any breast lumps in the past?
— Has anyone in your family had breast lumps?

Nipple discharge
— Do you have discharge from *both* nipples?
— What colour is the discharge?
— Have you breast-fed recently?

Hormonal factors
— Does the lump change with your menstrual cycle or at different times in the month?
— When did you start your periods? *(menarche)*
  If relevant, When did you stop your periods? *(menopause)*
— How many children do you have? Did you breast-feed them? Were there any problems?
— Have you ever been on the pill or hormone replacement therapy?

THE EXAMINATION

The usual instruction given in the short case is to "examine the breasts". Proceed as below.
Occasionally, you may be asked just to feel and describe a lump in the breast, in which case you should proceed as described on pages 20-23. Remember at all times to be sensitive and to avoid discomfort and embarrassment. Cover the breasts up when you are examining other systems.

"Examine this patient's breasts"

ACTION	NOTE
– Introduce yourself	
– Ask permission to examine the patient	
– Expose the breasts with the patient at 45° to the horizontal	

LOOK

ACTION	NOTE
– Stand opposite the patient	
– Ask her to raise her arms slowly above her head	*?asymmetry* *?nipple retraction* *?skin puckering*

FEEL

ACTION	NOTE
	If your patient has pendulous breasts, lie her flatter. Rest the arm of the breast to be examined behind her head. Ask her to lean slightly to the other side
– Ask the patient to point to the lump with one finger	
– Ask if the breasts are tender	
– Start with the normal breast Palpate *systematically*, each quadrant in turn and then centrally around the nipple Palpate with the flat of your fingers	

– Palpate the *affected* breast:
all quadrants except that of
the lump itself

– Try to elicit any discharge
by gently squeezing the nipple

colour: ?*red*
        ?*green*
        ?*yellow*
        ?*clear*
site: ?*nipple segment*

ASSESS THE LUMP

Omit this section if no lump is
found on examination

– *Feel* and *measure* the lump

overlying skin: ?*warm*

texture: ?*stony-hard*
        ?*rubbery-hard*
        ?*soft*

shape/size: ?*exact dimensions*

– Try to move the skin
overlying the lump

skin: ?*no movement* (implies
      fixation)

?*wrinkles at extremes
of movement* (implies
tethering)

– Ask your patient to rest her
hand lightly on the hip of the
same side. Move the lump
with your finger and thumb:
    • up and down
    • at right angles

?*mobility*

– Ask her to press hard on
her hip
Move the lump as above

movement of lump: ?*reduced on
contraction of pectoralis muscles*
(indicates attachment to muscle)

– Examine the axillae:
 hold the patient's right elbow
 in your right hand
 Take the weight of her forearm

– Palpate the walls:
 • medial
 • anterior
 • lateral
 • posterior
 • apical

If in doubt, palpate from
behind patient

?associated lymphadenopathy

– Repeat on the other side

– Palpate the cervical nodes

– Palpate the supraclavicular
 fossae and behind
 sternomastoid

ASSESS FURTHER

– Palpate the liver

?hepatomegaly
?knobbly edge
?tenderness

– Percuss down the back
 Ask if it is tender at any point
– Percuss the lung bases

?dull

**COMPLETE THE
EXAMINATION**

– Cover the patient's
 breasts with a sheet

– Turn to the examiner and
 present your findings

TYPICAL CASES

Breast lumps come up as long and short cases.
Revise the causes of a breast lump:

a. Physiological: Fibroadenosis

b. Neoplastic: (i) *Benign*   • Fibroadenoma
                                   • Duct papilloma
                                   • Phylloides tumour

              (ii) *Malignant*   • Primary carcinoma
                                  • Secondary carcinoma

c. Traumatic: Fat necrosis

d. Infective: Abscesses

You should be able to differentiate clinically between the commoner lumps:

	CARCINOMA	FIBROADENOMA	FIBROADENOSIS
No. of Lumps	1	1+	1+
Pain	rare	rare	common: varies with menstrual cycle
Irregularity	+ +	−	−
Hardness	+ + +	+ +	+

Case 1: *Breast carcinoma*

This is a very common case. Remember the classical features:

    (i) *Age 35+*

    (ii) *Positive family history*

    (iii) *Lump*: • Stony hard
                   • Irregular edge
                   • Tethered/fixed to skin *
                   • Immobile

    (iv) *Nipple*: • Inverted
                   • Distorted
                   • Peu d'orange
                   • Bloody discharge
                   • Red, encrusted, oozing (Paget's disease)

    (v) *Lymphadenopathy*

    (vi) *Features of metastases*: • Backache
                                   • Breathlessness
                                   • Jaundice
                                   • Malaise and weight loss

* *Note*: the differences between tethering and fixation:

	TETHERING	**FIXATION**
Infiltration	Along ligaments of Astley Cooper	To skin
Mobility	Some	None
Skin	Dimples at extremes of movement	Cannot be moved over lump
Prognosis	Better	Worse

Remember that the signs of breast carcinoma may be mimicked by other conditions. Consider the following:

(i)   *Hard irregular lumps*: fat necrosis and chronic mastitis.

(ii) *Nipple inversion*: this may be long-standing or congenital.

(iii) *Nipple discharge*: see Case 4.

(iv) *Nipple skin changes*: differentiate Paget's disease from eczema:

	PAGET'S DISEASE	**ECZEMA**
Cause	Spread of intraductal carcinoma to epidermis	Atopy
Bilateral?	No	Yes
Itchy?	No	Yes
Vesicular?	No	Yes

Case 2:   Fibroadenoma
A woman with a fibroadenoma will usually be young (peak 25-35).
There may be more than one lump. The lumps are small and rubbery-hard.
They are very mobile and are therefore also known as 'breast mice'.

Case 3:   Fibroadenosis
This condition is very common and borders on physiological change.
It occurs in women of reproductive age, peak 35-45. Ask specifically about variation with the menstrual cycle.

There are many presentations:
- Single lump (solid or cystic)
- Multiple lumps or generalised nodularity
- Cyclical breast pain
- Nipple discharge (clear, white or green)

Case 4: Nipple discharge

Ask yourself the following key questions:

a. Is the discharge true?

Eczema, Paget's disease and fistulae all cause discharges which do *not* arise from the ducts themselves.

b. Is the discharge significant?

For a discharge to be significant, it must have occurred:
- spontaneously
- over a year after stopping breast-feeding
- more than once

c. Is the discharge worrying?

The following features suggest carcinoma:
- *Unilateral* discharge
- *Bloody* discharge
- Discharge arising from a *single* duct (single nipple segment)

The colour of the discharge may give you a clue as to the cause:

COLOUR	NATURE	CAUSE
Red	Blood	• Ductal carcinoma • Duct papilloma
Green	Cell debris	• Fibroadenosis • Duct ectasia
Yellow	Exudate	• Fibroadenosis • Abscess
White	Milk	• Lactation

POPULAR VIVA QUESTIONS

— What are the presenting features of breast carcinoma?

— What do you understand by the term 'early breast cancer'?

— How would you manage a woman with early breast cancer?

— What is advanced breast cancer?

— What are the alternative treatments in advanced breast cancer?

— What are the advantages of mammography for breast cancer screening?

— What is Paget's disease of the nipple?

— What are the causes of nipple discharge?

— How does breast cancer spread?

— What are the advantages of lumpectomy over mastectomy for breast cancer?

— What benign breast diseases come into the differential diagnosis of breast cancer?

— What is a fibroadenoma?

— How may fibroadenosis present?

9: THE GASTROINTESTINAL TRACT

THE HISTORY

Give a succinct and chronological report of your patient's presenting complaint. Bring out the following aspects in your presentation:

The history of the patient's pain
(see page 19)

The history of the patient's lump/swelling
(see page 19)

Remainder of systemic enquiry of the GIT
Ask about the following symptoms:

- Dysphagia
- Dyspepsia
- Abdominal swelling/distension
- Nausea and vomiting
- Appetite and weight loss
- Change in bowel habit

Remember that diarrhoea/constipation are not precise words: ask what is normal for your patient.
Report on the stool:

?consistency
?frequency
?colour
?blood (?mixed in ?on the surface ?on the toilet paper)
?anal discharge/pruritus ani

THE EXAMINATION

Listen carefully to the instruction. In a short case, you may be asked to "examine the gastrointestinal system" or "examine the abdomen".
As with the examination of any system, always start with the hands. You may be stopped at this stage and asked to proceed to the abdomen itself.
Occasionally, you may be instructed to "palpate the abdomen", in which case beginning with the hands will only antagonise the examiners.

Note the following points:

● Make sure your hands are warm.

● Don't hurt your patient: during palpation, keep looking at his/her face for wincing.

● Don't forget the following parts on account of exam nerves:

    • Percussion of the upper border of the liver (*normally 5th intercostal space: may be displaced downwards with hyperexpansion of the chest*)
    • Groin
    • External genitalia
    • Statement that you would normally perform a rectal examination

Also remember the **3 As**:

    • Aortic aneurysm
    • Ascites
    • Auscultation

"Examine this patient's gastrointestinal system"

ACTION	NOTE
– Introduce yourself	
– Ask permission to examine the patient	
– Expose the abdomen with the patient lying flat with one pillow supporting the head	Include the inguinal regions but not the genitalia

I. PRELIMINARY ASSESSMENT

– Look at both hands	nails: *?clubbing* *?leuconychia* palms: *?palmar erythema* *?Dupuytren's contracture* *?pallor of skin creases*
– Ask patient to stretch out arms with the wrists cocked up	*?liver flap*
– Look at the eyes	sclera: *?jaundice* conjunctiva: *?pallor*
– Look at the mouth	*?telangiectasia* (indicates hereditary haemorrhagic telangiectasia) *?perioral pigmentation* (indicates Peutz-Jegher's syndrome)

– Ask patient to stick out tongue	*?dehydration* *?coated tongue*
– Smell breath	*?ketosis* *?halitosis*
– Palpate cervical lymph nodes	In this case, it is not necessary to examine from behind the patient *?cervical lymphadenopathy*
– Show the examiner you are paying particular attention to the *left* supraclavicular fossa	*?Virchow's node/Troisier's sign*
– Look at the chest	skin: *?spider naevi* *?purpura*
– Feel gently around the nipples	*?gynaecomastia*

II. THE ABDOMEN

LOOK

– Stand at the end of the bed
Ask patient to take a deep breath, draw in the abdomen and cough
	skin: *?scars*
	       ?stoma site
	       ?visible veins
	shape: *?distended*
	       ?scaphoid
	       ?visible peristalis
	       ?visible masses

FEEL

Palpate with your palm and the flat of your fingers Keep your forearm level with the abdominal wall	You may need to kneel down if the bed is low

a. <u>Preliminary palpation</u>

− Ask if the abdomen is tender
− Palpate each quadrant *lightly*

?*tenderness*
?*guarding*
?*rigidity*

− Palpate each quadrant more
deeply, leaving the tender
areas until last

?*deep tenderness*
?*masses*
?*palpable viscera*

b. <u>Assessment of a mass</u>

− If you find a mass, determine
its characteristics at this
stage (pages 20-23)

?*size*
?*shape*
?*surface*
?*edge*
?*consistency*
?*percussion note*
?*bruit/bowel sounds*

c. <u>Assessment of organomegaly</u>

(i) *Liver*

− Palpate the liver, beginning
in the right iliac fossa
As patient breathes in and
out, move your hand upwards
in stages until you reach the
costal margin

?*hepatomegaly*
?*smooth edge*
?*knobbly edge*
?*consistency*
?*tenderness*
?*pulsatility*

− Percuss out the liver: lower
and upper borders

?*dull*

(ii) *Spleen*

– Palpate the spleen, beginning
in the right iliac fossa   ?*splenomegaly*
As patient breathes in and out,
move your hand towards tip
of the tenth rib
On reaching the costal margin,   If you still cannot feel the
place your left hand around   spleen, ask the patient to
the lower left rib cage   roll towards you
Palpate with your right hand
in the midaxillary line

– Percuss for an enlarged spleen   ?*dull*

(iii) *Kidneys*

– Palpate each kidney: position   Your hand should be *well*
one hand behind patient's loin   behind patient's loin
and the other hand just
above ASIS
Ask patient to breath deeply   ?*enlarged kidneys*

(iv) *Aortic aneurysm*

– Place two hands along the   ?*expansile pulsation*
midline, just above the
umblilicus

d. Examination of groin and
   external genitalia

– Place your fingers over the   ?*cough impulse*
inguinal and femoral orifices
Ask patient to cough

– Feel inguinal lymph nodes   ?*inguinal lymphadenopathy*

– Feel testes   ?*atrophy*
                                  ?*mass*

e. Examination for ascites

This is only necessary if the abdomen is distended

(i) *Shifting dullness*

– Percuss over the abdomen Start centrally and move to the flanks

Keep your finger in the sagittal plane

– Locate the point on one side where the percussion note changes from resonant to dull

– Ask patient to roll over on that side, keeping your hand in this position

– Percuss again

?has area of dullness moved

(ii) *Fluid thrill*

– Ask patient to place the edge of his/her hand along the midline

– Flick one side while feeling the other side

?thrill

LISTEN

– Auscultate abdomen over at least three different areas

bowel sounds: *?pitch*

– Listen along the course of the aorta and iliac arteries and in the renal areas

?bruits

SAY

"I would like to:
• do a rectal examination
• examine the urine with a dipstick"

?mass
?proteinuria
?haematuria
?glucose

**COMPLETE THE
EXAMINATION**

– Cover the patient up

– Turn to the examiner

– Present your findings

TYPICAL CASES

You are unlikely to meet a patient with an 'acute abdomen' in either the short or long case. However, you should revise the causes of acute abdominal pain for discussion in the clinical examination and viva.

In the long case, you may meet patients with abdominal symptoms but few signs. Examples are patients with *peptic ulcers*, *chronic cholecystitis* (and bouts of *biliary colic*), *chronic pancreatitis*, *diverticular disease*, *irritable bowel syndrome* and *inflammatory bowel disease*.

You may also have a patient with *jaundice*. In a surgical examination, the most likely cause will be post-hepatic 'obstructive' jaundice. However, when asked the differential diagnosis, mention pre-hepatic and hepatocellular causes.

The main physical signs, to be picked up in both the long and short case, are scars and stomas, organomegaly, masses and distension. This section revises the differential diagnosis of these signs.

I. SCARS AND STOMAS

Scars

Always look very carefully for abdominal scars: old ones are surprisingly easy to miss, especially in hirsute men. It is particularly easy to miss a Pfannenstiel incision, appendicectomy scar and a left nephrectomy scar (look well over the left loin).

You should know the usual sites:

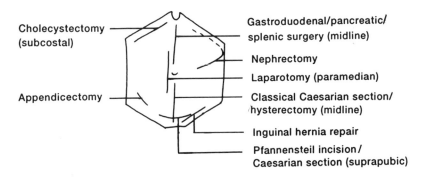

Cholecystectomy (subcostal)

Gastroduodenal/pancreatic/splenic surgery (midline)

Nephrectomy

Laparotomy (paramedian)

Appendicectomy

Classical Caesarian section/hysterectomy (midline)

Inguinal hernia repair

Pfannensteil incision/Caesarian section (suprapubic)

Stomas

You should understand the differences between ileostomies and colostomies:

	ILEOSTOMY	COLOSTOMY
Type	Permanent only	Temporary or permanent
Indications	• Ulcerative colitis; Crohn's disease • Inherited polyposis coli	• Colorectal carcinoma • Diverticular disease
Appearance	Spout of mucosa	Mucosa sutured to skin
Position	Right iliac fossa	• Permanent: left iliac fossa • Temporary: right hypochondrium or left iliac fossa
Effluent	Continuous	Intermittent
Complications	Fluid and electrolyte imbalance • Ischaemia • Obstruction • Skin erosion • Recurrent disease at stoma site • Bowel prolapse • Parastomal hernia	

II. ORGANOMEGALY

Case 1: *Hepatomegaly*

In a surgical examination, the most common cause of hepatomegaly is metastases. The patient may or may not be jaundiced. Your examiner will expect you to know the other causes of hepatomegaly.

Common causes in the United Kingdom include the following:
- Metastases
- Congestive cardiac failure (right sided)
- Cirrhosis (not in later stages, when liver shrinks and is impalpable)
- Infections, eg viral hepatitis, infectious mononucleosis

Go through your surgical seive (page 12) to retrieve rarer causes.

Your *description* of the liver should help in your differential diagnosis:

a. Edge: (i) *Smooth*   • Cirrhosis
                              • Congestive heart failure

            (ii) *Knobbly*   • Secondary carcinoma
                              • Macronodular cirrhosis (rare)

b. Consistency: *Hard* if metastases

c. Tenderness: Occurs when capsule is distended:
                              • Congestive heart failure
                              • Hepatitis
                              • Hepatocellular carcinoma
                              • AV malformation
                              • Alcoholic hepatitis (rare)

d. Pulsatility: • Tricuspid regurgitation

Case 2: Splenomegaly

If your patient has splenomegaly, you may well be asked to justify your diagnosis in terms of its five distinguishing characteristics:

- Descends towards the right iliac fossa
- Moves down on inspiration
- Palpable medial notch
- Cannot get above it
- Dull to percussion (continuous with area of splenic dullness over 9th, 10th and 11th ribs, behind posterior axillary line)

Have a list of causes of massive, moderate and mild splenomegaly. As always, give the common causes in the UK first (eg myelofibrosis rather than kala-azar, for massive splenomegaly).

MASSIVE	MODERATE	MILD
	As for massive *plus*	As for moderate *plus*
• Myelofibrosis	• Haemolytic anaemia	• Infectious mononucleosis
• Chronic Granulocytic Leukaemia	• Chronic lymphocytic leukaemia	• Myleoproliferative disorders
• Malaria	• Lymphomas	• Pernicious anaemia
• Kala-azar	• Portal hypertension	• Amyloidosis
		• Sarcoidosis
		• Rheumatoid arthritis (Felty's syndrome)

Although many of these causes of splenomegaly are 'medical', your patient may be awaiting a splenectomy because of its complications: *hypersplenism* would lead to both pooling and destruction by the reticulo-endothelial system of haemopoietic cells, causing a pancytopaenia. Be aware of the potential problems of splenectomy, eg infection with capsulated bacteria such as pneumococcus. Know about the measures to reduce such complications (pneumovax immunization, prophylactic penicillin).

Case 3: *Hepatosplenomegaly*
Causes of enlargement of the spleen as well as the liver include some of the above, eg lymphoma, leukaemias, infections, amyloidosis and sarcoidosis. The most likely case in an examination is cirrhosis with associated portal hypertension.

Case 4: *Enlarged kidneys*
Remember that in slim people, the lower pole of the right kidney may be palpable.
Know the characteristics of a renal swelling:

- Ballottable *(bimanually palpable)*
- Descends vertically
- Moves down on respiration
- Resonant to percussion due to overlying colon *(not always*: some parts may be dull)
- Can get above it *(rarely)*

Another popular question is to differentiate between an enlarged left kidney and a palpable spleen:

	KIDNEY	**SPLEEN**
Descent on inspiration?	Vertically	Towards right iliac fossa
Ballottable?	Yes	No
Notch present?	No	Yes
Can you ever get above it?	Occasionally	No
Percussion note?	Resonant (usually)	Dull

In finals, the most common cause of *bilateral* renal enlargement is polycystic kidneys. These may be extremely large and feel lobulated because of the multiple cysts. If you suspect this condition,

— Ask about family history (inheritence is *autosomal dominant*).
— Take the blood pressure.
— Ask to examine the urine (*?haematuria ?proteinuria ?casts*).
— Try to palpate a liver which may also be polycystic.
— Look for a third nerve palsy due to pressure from an associated posterior communicating artery Berry aneurysm.

Other causes of bilateral renal enlargement are bilateral hydronephrosis and amyloidosis.

Causes of *unilateral* renal enlargement include the following:
• Hydronephrosis
• Simple benign cysts
• Hypertrophy
• Tumour, eg renal cell carcinoma

A transplanted kidney will usually be found in an iliac fossa.

III. MASSES

Revise pages 20-23 for the description of any mass.
As many masses are visible on careful observation of the abdomen, do not forget to *look* first.
List and revise the causes of masses in each segment of the abdomen.

Case 5: *Mass in right hypochondrium*

The causes of a mass in the right hypondrium include the following:

- Hepatomegaly
- Enlarged gallbladder
- Enlarged right kidney
- Colonic mass

Revise the causes of an enlarged gallbladder:

(i)   *Obstruction of cystic duct*: mucocoele or empyema.

(ii) *Obstuction of the common bile duct*, eg cancer of the head of the pancreas.

Remember *Courvoisier's law*:

"If the gallbladder is palpable and the patient is jaundiced, the obstruction of the bile duct causing the jaundice is unlikely to be due to a stone."

(iii) *Gallbladder mass*: inflammation with surrounding adherent omentum.

Also note the characteristics of an enlarged gallbladder:

- Appcars from the tip of the 9th rib
- Cannot get between it and the liver edge
- Dull to percussion
- Smooth surface
- Moves down on inspiration (not always true of gallbladder mass)

Case 6: Mass in epigastrium

The two most important causes are carcinoma of the stomach and pancreatic masses (pseudocyst, carcinoma).

Two 'catches' are:

(i) *Liver*: either left lobe or a post-necrotic nodule of a cirrhotic liver.

(ii) *Large recti*: these appear to enlarge when the patient sits forwards.

You should suspect gastric or pancreatic carcinoma in a cachectic patient complaining of pain, dyspepsia, anorexia and significant weight loss. You may not always feel a mass.

Note the characteristics of a *gastric* carcinoma:

- Hard, irregular
- Cannot get above it
- Moves with respiration

Think immediately of checking for a left supraclavicular node *(Virchow's node/Troisier's sign)*.

Gastric carcinoma may be difficult to differentiate from a pancreatic pseudocyst which, although uncommon, crops up disproportionately in examinations. The characteristics of a pancreatic pseudocyst are as follows:

- Cannot get above it
- Indistinct lower border
- Resonant to percussion
- Moves slightly with respiration

Case 7: Mass in left hypochondrium

The most common cause is an enlarged spleen. Other causes are a pancreatic mass (carcinoma of tail) and an enlarged left kidney.

Case 8: Right loin	*Case 9:* Umbilical region	*Case 10:* Left loin
• Enlarged right kidney	• Small bowel mass (nodal or omental)	• Enlarged left kidney
• Enlarged liver	• Cancer of transverse colon	• Enlarged spleen
• Enlarged gall bladder	• Aortic aneurysm	

Case 11: Mass in right iliac fossa

A mass in the right iliac fossa is a common clinical case.
The most common causes are carcinoma of the caecum and Crohn's disease.

a. Carcinoma of caecum

Suspect this condition in an elderly patient who appears clinically anaemic. The mass is often well-defined and hard. It may be mobile or fixed. It is not usually tender.

b. Crohn's disease

This is usually seen in younger patients. The mass feels rubbery and non-tender and may be fairly mobile.

These are the less common causes:
  • Appendix mass
  • Ileocaecal TB
  • Iliac lymphadenopathy
  • Ovarian cyst
  • Pelvic (transplanted) kidney

Case 12: Mass in left iliac fossa

The common causes are a loaded sigmoid colon (may be normally palpable, but particularly with constipation or diverticular disease) and carcinoma of the colon. Rarer causes are Crohn's disease and iliac lymphadenopathy. Again, don't forget gynaecological causes (eg an ovarian mass) or pelvic (transplanted) kidneys.

a. Diverticular disease

You are unlikely to be given a patient with a diverticular abscess.
However, patients with diverticular disease often have a palpable, tender sigmoid colon.

b. Carcinoma of colon

The patient normally presents with a change in bowel habit. The mass will usually be hard.
Feel for an enlarged liver and listen for high-pitched bowel sounds (in the presence of any obstruction).

Case 13: Suprapubic mass

Suprapubic masses are easily missed.

The two characteristics of a pelvic swelling are:
- • Cannot get below it
- • May be palpated bimanually on vaginal or rectal examination

The most common cause is an enlarged bladder. This has the following characteristics:
- • Dull to percussion
- • Fluid thrill
- • Direct pressure produces desire to micturate

In the female, do not forget the important gynaecological causes: the pregnant uterus, a large ovarian cyst and uterine fibroids.

In a surgical examination, you should express the importance of doing a vaginal examination to enable bimanual palpation. However, it is unlikely you will be asked to do so.

Case 14: Abdominal distension
Remember the **5 Fs**:

a. <u>Fe</u>tus: very unlikely in a surgical examination but always consider in a woman of reproductive age.

b. <u>Fl</u>atus: the abdomen will be hyper-resonant; you may see visible peristalsis.

c. <u>Fa</u>eces: you are unlikely to be given a patient with acute obstuction. However, chronic constipation is a common surgical problem. Beware - your patient may be complaining of diarrhoea and in fact be constipated (spurious diarrhoea).

   Faeces have the following characteristics:

   - Lie in the distribution of the colon
   - Often form multiple separate masses
   - Can be indented with digital pressure

d. <u>Fat</u>: usually obvious; deposition is in the lower half of the abdomen.

e. <u>Fl</u>uid: ascites can be detected by two tests: fluid thrill and shifting dullness. The latter is more reliable because a fluid thrill is detected in *any* abdominal fluid-filled cavity.

POPULAR VIVA QUESTIONS

— What are the causes of:

- dysphagia
- hepatomegaly
- splenomegaly
- hepatosplenomegaly
- jaundice
- change in bowel habit
- diarrhoea
- constipation
- blood PR
- haematemesis
- melaena
- intestinal obstruction: *?in children ?in adults*

— What are the complications of diverticular disease?

— What is the difference between diverticulosis and diverticulitis?

— What are the differences between Crohn's Disease and ulcerative colitis?

— What are the local and general complications of inflammatory bowel disease?

— How does presentation of carcinoma of the head of the pancreas differ from that of the tail of the pancreas?

— What is Dukes' staging for colorectal cancer?

— How does the presentation of carcinoma of the right side of the bowel differ from that of the left?

— How do gallstones present?

— What is the difference between peritonism and peritonitis?

— What are the symptoms of intestinal obstruction?

— What are the extra-abdominal causes of acute abdominal pain?

— Differentiate between tenderness, rebound tenderness, guarding and rigidity.

THE HISTORY

Hernias and groin lumps are very popular short cases. After examining a hernia, you may be instructed to ask the patient some additional questions. Structure them as follows:

The lump itself
(see page 19)

Predisposing causes
— Do you have a chronic cough/asthma/bronchitis?
— Do you do much heavy lifting?
— Do you have to strain to pass a motion?
  (Note that this may occur both with constipation and diarrhoea.)
— Do you have difficulty passing water?

Potential complications (strangulation and obstruction)
— Does the lump become tender or painful?
— Do you have any abdominal pain?
— Have you vomited recently?
— Have you noticed your abdomen swelling/your clothes getting tighter?
— Are you constipated?

THE EXAMINATION

In a short case, you may be asked specifically to "examine this hernia" or "this scrotal lump", in which case you should examine as for any lump (pages 20-23) plus perform the additional assessment outlined below. If you are asked to "examine the groin", follow the whole examination scheme.

Note the following points:

- You may see an inguinal lump you are certain is a hernia. However, always examine the scrotum as well. There may be dual pathology.

- Always examine both sides: **20%** of hernias are bilateral.

- Try to distinguish between a direct and an indirect inguinal hernia. Some say that this is unimportant as it does not affect the patient's management. However, you cannot be faulted for being too thorough.

"Examine this patient's groin"

ACTION	NOTE
– Introduce yourself	
– Ask permission to examine the patient	If there is an *obvious* inguino-scrotal swelling, do not stand the patient up. Otherwise, examine with the patient standing
– Expose the groin and external genitalia	

I. EXAMINATION OF THE EXTERNAL GENITALIA

LOOK

– Observe the anterior aspect of the scrotum	skin: ?*colour* swelling: ?*inguinal* ?*scrotal*
– Observe the posterior aspect of the scrotum, pulling on posterior skin, *not* the testes	

FEEL

– Roll the testes *gently* between your thumb (in front) and index finger (behind)	*?both testes palpable*
– Locate the epididymis (above and posterior to testis)	*?epididymal swelling*
– Feel along the spermatic cord	*?cord swelling*

ASSESSMENT OF SWELLING

– Define its characteristics (see pages 20-23)	*?size* *?shape* *?fluctuant* *?transilluminable*
– Try to locate its upper edge	*?can you get above it*
– Try to feel testis	*?testis separate from swelling*

II. EXAMINATION FOR HERNIAS

– Stand to one side of the patient who should be standing Locate the pubic tubercle Place one hand behind patient and the examining hand over the swelling	If no swelling is seen, place your hand over the superficial ring (just above and medial to the pubic tubercle)

ASSESS THE SWELLING

– Define its characteristics (see pages 20-23)	*?size* *?shape* *?fluctuant* *?transilluminable*

– Press firmly over the
swelling/superficial ring

– Ask patient to turn his/her
head away from you and cough   *?expansile cough impulse*

– Ask patient to try and   He/she may request to lie
reduce the hernia   down to do this

– While the hernia is still
reduced, place two fingers
over the deep ring (half-way
between pubic tubercle
and ASIS)

– Ask patient to cough
Watch

– Release the pressure   *?hernia controlled by*
                                pressure over deep ring
                                (indicates indirect hernia)

– Go to the other side of patient
Repeat the examination

**COMPLETE THE
EXAMINATION**

– Cover the patient up

– Turn to the examiner

– Ask to wash your hands

– Present your findings

TYPICAL CASES

I. INGUINAL SWELLINGS AND HERNIAS

One way to remember the differential diagnosis of lumps in the groin is to think of the structures that normally lie in the region.

(i) *Hernias*
- Inguinal (direct, indirect)
- Femoral

(ii) *Vascular structures*
- Saphena varix
- Femoral aneurysm

(iii) *Lymph nodes*
- Lymphadenopathy

(iv) *Muscle*
- Psoas abscess

(v) *Testis*
- Ectopic testis (in superficial inguinal pouch)
- Undescended testis (as it emerges from superficial ring)

(vi) *Spermatic cord*
- Lipoma of the cord
- Hydrocoele of the cord

Have a clear picture of the relation of these structures to the inguinal ligament:

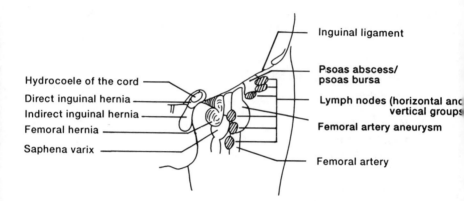

You may be asked what is meant by the term 'hernia'. The definition should roll off your tongue:
"The protrusion of the whole or part of a viscus, from its normal position, through an opening in the wall of its containing cavity".

Another common question is: "Why must a hernia be repaired?"
The answer is because of the potential complications of *obstruction* and *strangulation*. You should understand exactly what is meant by these two terms:

> *Obstruction*: constriction at the neck of a hernial sac leads to obstruction of the loops of bowel within it.

> *Strangulation*: constriction prevents venous return causing venous congestion, arterial occlusion and gangrene. This may lead to perforation causing peritonitis or a groin abscess.

Note that strangulation may occur without obstruction if only one wall of a viscus pouches into the sac ('Richter's hernia').

Case 1: *Inguinal hernia*

There is not much anatomy you need to know for finals.
However, a favourite question is to describe the anatomy of the inguinal canal: this is an intermuscular oblique passage 4cm long. The following structures pass through it:

- Spermatic cord/round ligament
- Ilioinguinal nerve

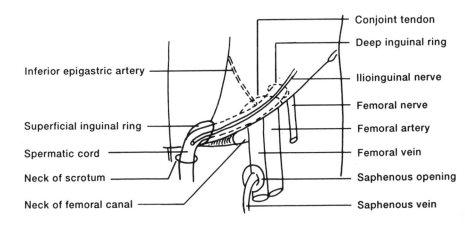

a. The walls

	ANTERIOR	**POSTERIOR**	**FLOOR**	**ROOF**
Medially	External oblique	Conjoint tendon	Inguinal ligament + Lacunar ligament	Conjoint tendon
Laterally	External + Internal oblique	Fascia transversalis	Inguinal ligament	

b. The rings

(i)   *External Ring*
This is formed by the two crura of the external oblique aponeurosis. It lies just above and medial to the pubic tubercle.

(ii)   *Internal Ring*
This is a U-shaped condensation of the fascia transversalis.
It lies at the mid-point of the inguinal ligament. The inferior epigastric artery (branch of external iliac) runs *medially*.

Note the difference between the *mid-point of the inguinal ligament* (half-way between the ASIS and the pubic tubercle) and the *mid-inguinal point* (half-way between the ASIS and the pubic symphysis - landmark of the femoral pulse). The mid-point of the inguinal ligament lies 1-1.5cm lateral to the mid-inguinal point.

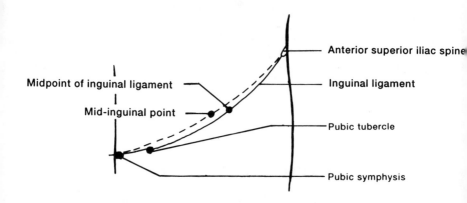

Understand the anatomy of direct and indirect hernias:

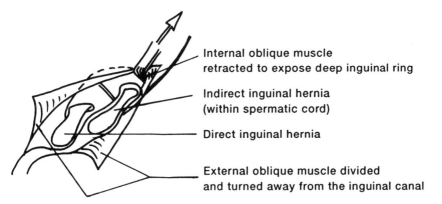

Internal oblique muscle
retracted to expose deep inguinal ring

Indirect inguinal hernia
(within spermatic cord)

Direct inguinal hernia

External oblique muscle divided
and turned away from the inguinal canal

Some examiners are keen for you to be able to distinguish clinically between
a direct and indirect hernia:

	DIRECT	**INDIRECT**
Extends to scrotum?	No	Yes
Direction of reduction	Straight back	Up and lateral
Controlled by pressure over internal ring?	No	Yes
Direction of reappearance after reduction	To original position	Down and medial

Case 2: Femoral hernia

You should know how to distinguish clinically a femoral from an inguinal hernia:

	INGUINAL HERNIA	FEMORAL HERNIA
Position relative to pubic tubercle	Superior and medial	Inferior and lateral *
Palpation	Soft	Firm: like bouncing a ball underwater
Percussion	May be resonant	Dull
Auscultation	Bowel sounds commonly heard	Bowel sounds rarely heard

* *Note*: Femoral hernias may bulge up into the groin crease (as shown on page 96).

Note the following additional points:

- In both men and women inguinal hernias are more common than femoral hernias. However, femoral hernias are more common in females than males.

- A femoral hernia is more likely to obstruct and strangulate than an inguinal hernia because of the narrow femoral ring. Furthermore, a femoral hernia is more likely than an inguinal hernia to strangulate without obstructing (Richter's hernia).

Revise the anatomy of the femoral canal:

Medially: lacunar ligament
Laterally: femoral vein
Supero-anteriorly: inguinal ligament
Infero-posteriorly: pectineal ligament of Astley Cooper

The table below gives some of the clinical feature of some other inguinal swellings.

	CONSISTENCY	COMPRESS-IBILITY?	COUGH IMPULSE?	OTHER FEATURES
Case 3: **Saphena varix**	Very soft	Yes	Yes	• Fluid thrill • Varicose veins
Case 4: **Femoral aneurysm**	Firm	No	No	• Expansile pulsation • Bruit
Case 5: **Lymph node**	Hard	No	No	• *Multiple* nodules • *Generalised* lymphadeno-pathy
Case 6: **Psoas abscess**	Soft	Yes	No	• Fluctuation between parts of abscess above and below inguinal ligament

II. SCROTAL AND INGUINOSCROTAL SWELLINGS

It is unlikely you will be given a patient with a very tender swelling in an examination as this usually implies the following:

- Torsion of the testis: a surgical emergency
- Severe epididymo-orchitis: rare

A simplified diagnostic flowchart which excludes the latter two conditions is given below:

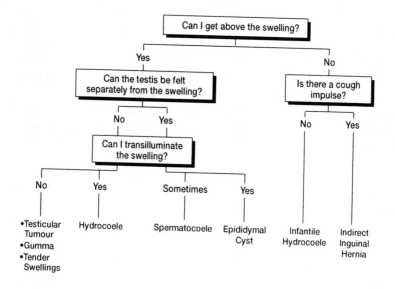

Case 7: *Testicular tumour*

This is an opaque mass, not felt discretely from the testis. It is usually painless but occasionally causes a dull ache.

Remember that it may be associated with a secondary hydrocoele.

Note that lymphatic spread is along the site of its embryological origin, ie to para-aortic lymph nodes. It only spreads to inguinal nodes if the scrotum is invaded.

Case 8: *Varicocoele*

This is a dilatation and elongation of the Pampiniform plexus of veins, usually found on the left.

It is said to feel like a 'bag of worms'.

It can only be felt with the patient standing.

Case 9: *Hydrocoele*

This is a swelling that cannot be felt separately from the testis. It is fluctuant and transilluminable. It is due to excessive fluid collecting in the tunica vaginalis.

Understand the anatomy of the four types of hydrocoele. All of these come into your differential diagnosis of inguinal and inguino-scrotal lumps. A vaginal hydrocoele is by far the most common.

TYPE	AGE	COMMUNI-CATION WITH PERITONEAL CAVITY?	NOTE	DIAGRAM
a. Vaginal	All	No	May be *secondary* to underlying infection or a testicular tumour	
b. Congenital	Child (aged < 3 yrs)	Yes	Main differential diagnosis is an indirect inguinal hernia: communicating orifice is too small for hernia to develop	
c. Infantile	All	No	Due to incomplete reabsorption of fluid from the tunica vaginalis after the processus vaginalis seals off	
d. Encysted hydrocoele of the cord	All	No	May occur anywhere along cord, causing a scrotal *or* inguinal lump	

Case 10: *Epididymal cyst*

Like a hydrocoele, this is brilliantly transilluminable. However, the testis *can* be felt separately.

Note that if it is filled with many sperm, it may be opaque. In this case, it is called a *spermatocoele*.

Case 11: *Absent testis in a child*

Put your hand just lateral to the external ring and apply firm pressure downwards and medially. If you can 'milk' the testis down into the scrotum, the testis is *retractile*: descent is normal, but excessive cremasteric muscle activity in young children leads to the testis being drawn up.

Look carefully for other swellings in the area; there may be an *ectopic* testis. You may feel a lump in the following positions:

- Superficial inguinal pouch (superficial to external oblique and lateral to the pubic tubercle)
- Femoral canal (medial thigh)
- Perianally

Once you have *excluded* retractile and ectopic testes, you may diagnose an incompletely descended testis.

Remember to search for an inguinal hernia. This is present in 90% of cases of incompletely descended testes.

POPULAR VIVA QUESTIONS

— Define 'hernia'.

— Where might you find a hernia, other than the groin?

— What factors can predispose to inguinal hernias?

— What are the surface markings of the superficial inguinal ring/the deep inguinal ring?

— Describe the anatomy of the inguinal/femoral canal.

— Why do we repair hernias?

— What are the complications of hernias?

— What is the difference between an indirect and a direct inguinal hernia?

— Define the terms, 'herniotomy' and 'herniorrhaphy'.

— What is the treatment of a strangulated inguinal hernia?

— How would you manage a patient with a testicular tumour?

THE HISTORY

'Arteriopath' patients are readily available for examinations because of their age and complications. They are usually given as long cases, as the histories tend to be extensive. In your 'history of presenting complaint', include not only the symptoms of peripheral vascular disease, but also all other symptoms, risk factors, past history and family history of cardiovascular and cerebrovascular disease:

Presenting symptoms:

— Can you describe the pain in your legs? *(Ask pain questions, see page 19)*

— Does the pain come on when you walk/exercise?

— How far can you walk before you get the pain? (Claudication distance is best described in terms of a *known* distance, eg from the entrance of the hospital to the clinic.)

— When you stop walking, how long does it take for the pain to go away?

— Can you walk *through* the pain?

— How long have you had the problem? Has it got any better or worse over this time?

— How does it affect your lifestyle?

— Have you any pain in your leg or foot at rest?

— What relieves your pain? (Rest pain may be relieved by walking about and hanging the leg over the side of the bed.)

In a man, ask about erectile function (Leriche's syndrome).

Past surgical history

Ask about past operations and investigations for peripheral vascular disease. When you present your history, describe these events chronologically and as concisely as possible.

Past medical history

Ask about previous myocardial infarcts / strokes / transient ischaemic attacks.

Associated cardiovascular and cerebrovascular problems

Ask about chest pain / shortness of breath on exertion / palpitations / ankle swelling.

Risk factors

Ask about smoking / cholesterol levels / hypertension / diabetes.

Family history

Ask about a family history of cardiovascular / cerebrovascular / peripheral vascular disease.

Tailor the rest of your history towards the differential diagnosis. For example, it is important to ask about neurological symptoms, eg paraesthesia in the leg, as there may be a neurological cause of the pain.

THE EXAMINATION

The long case

Pay particular attention to the following:

- Peripheral vascular system: look for ulcers on pressure areas and over the tips and between the toes. Record all pulses and bruits on a diagram (see page 111).

- Heart

- Fundoscopy

- Neurological examination of the lower limb: in a patient complaining of leg pain, you may be asked to explain how your examination findings point to a diagnosis of claudication/rest pain rather than nerve root pain.

The short case

Listen carefully to the instruction: if your examiner asks you to examine the patient's *lower limb*, do not jump straight into the following scheme, but follow the systematic approach outlined on page 180. Similarly, if asked to examine an ulcer on a limb, proceed as for the examination of any ulcer (pages 24-25).

"Examine this patient's peripheral vascular system"

ACTION	NOTE
– Introduce yourself	
– Ask permission to examine the patient	
– Expose both legs completely	
LOOK	
– Stand at the end of the bed and observe	Colour: *?white/blue/black*
	Trophic changes: *?shiny skin* *?hair loss* *?loss of subcutaneous tissue* *?ulcers*
– Look at pressure points: • lateral side of foot • head of 1st metatarsal • heel • malleoli	Ulcers: *?size* (pages 24-25) *?shape/dimensions* *?depth* *?edge* *?base*
– Observe: • tips of toes • between toes	

FEEL

– Run the back of your
  hand along both limbs
  Compare both sides

?warm/cold
?point of temperature change

– Press the tip of a nail
  for two seconds
  Count the number of
  seconds for the nail to
  become pink again

?capillary refilling time

– Feel pulses:

Compare right with left
In the long case, use a
diagram to record pulses and
bruits:

a. Femoral pulse: feel
midway between symphysis
pubis and ASIS (mid-inguinal
point)

b. Popliteal pulse: ask the
patient to bend his/her knee
Put your thumbs on the tibial
tuberosity and feel pulse
with eight finger tips

c. Dorsalis pedis: feel along
cleft between first two
metatarsals
Use three fingers

d. Posterior tibial: half-way
along line between medial
malleolus and the prominence
of the heel

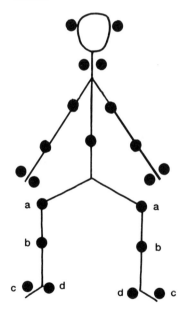

LISTEN

– Listen for bruits at all
  sites, ie along iliac,
  femoral and popliteal
  arteries on both sides

ASSESS FURTHER

– Elevate leg about 15°
  Look

?venous guttering

– Elevate leg further

*?angle at which leg becomes
  pale* (Buerger's angle)

– Then ask patient to hang
  leg over side of bed
  (Buerger's test)

*?time of venous filling
?reactive hyperaemia on
  dependency*

SAY

"I would like to
examine:
• the rest of the
  peripheral vascular
  system
• the heart
• the abdomen for an
  aortic aneurysm"

If asked to assess rest of peripheral vascular system,

- Feel:
  - radial pulse
  - carotid pulse

- Listen for:
  - carotid bruit
    (just behind angle of mandible)
  - subclavian bruit
  - radio-femoral delay

COMPLETE THE EXAMINATION

- Make sure your patient is comfortable

- Cover the legs

- Turn to your examiner and present your findings

TYPICAL CASES

It is extremely unlikely that you will have a patient with an acutely ischaemic limb in the examination, as this is a surgical emergency. However, be aware of the causes of acute ischaemia and the symptoms and signs - remember the **6 P's: P**ain, **P**araesthesia, **P**aralysis, **P**allor, **P**ulselessness, **P**erishingly cold.

Case 1: Intermittent claudication

Don't worry if your history doesn't fit into any neat catagory: just report clearly and confidently on your findings. Ask yourself the following questions; this will help enormously in your presentation and discussion of the case with the examiners:

a. <u>Is your patient's pain due to vascular disease?</u>

It is quite possible that your patient has symptomless arterial disease with loss of pulses, but is suffering from a different cause of leg pain. Know the features of claudication pain:

- Cramp-like
- Felt in the muscle
- Comes on invariably and only with exercise
- Stops after about two minutes of rest

b. <u>What is the differential diagnosis?</u>

Think of the following:

(i) *Sciatica*

This is differentiated from claudication by the following features:

- History of disc lesion/back trouble
- Pain felt in back, down buttock and thigh
- No characteristic relationship to exercise
- Limited straight leg raising
- Neurological signs, eg wasting, loss of power, reflexes and sensation

(ii) *Osteoarthritis of the hip*

This can be difficult to distinguish as the pain is also worsened by exercise
The pain is felt in the hip joint but may be referred to the knee.
It varies from day to day.

(iii) *Anterior tibial compartment syndrome* (rare in an examination)

This occurs in young people after unaccustomed exercise. The pain is felt
in the *anterior* part of the lower leg.

(iv) *Cauda equina claudication*

This is the most difficult to distinguish. There are two pathologies. Both
lead to sciatic-like pain and to limited straight leg raising after exercise.

- Disc pathology: partial compression of cauda equina by prolapsed
  disc.
- Aorto-iliac disease: on exercise, a drop in pressure leads to
  ischaemia of cauda equina.

c. <u>What is the site of the main occlusion?</u>

Try to relate your patient's symptoms (site of pain) and signs (absence of pulses, presence of bruits) to the anatomy. A mental picture of the angiogram helps:

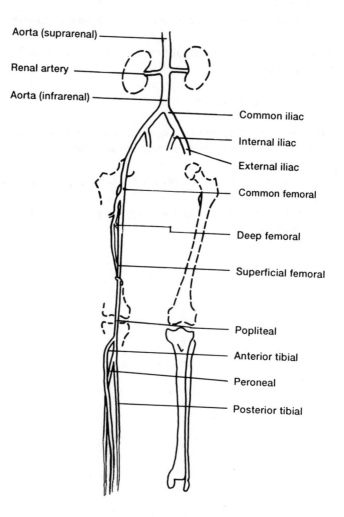

Aorta (suprarenal)

Renal artery

Aorta (infrarenal)

Common iliac

Internal iliac

External iliac

Common femoral

Deep femoral

Superficial femoral

Popliteal

Anterior tibial

Peroneal

Posterior tibial

Distinguish between femoro-distal disease and aorto-iliac disease:

	FEMORO-DISTAL DISEASE	**AORTO-ILIAC DISEASE**
Site of pain	• Calf	• Calf • Thigh • Buttock
Absent pulses	• Foot • Popliteal	• Foot • Popliteal • Femoral

If aorto-iliac symptoms are unilateral, occlusion is probably of the common iliac artery. If symptoms are bilateral (rare), occlusion may be of the aorta. Think of the tetrad of Leriche's syndrome:
- Bilateral pain
- Impotence in male (no flow in internal iliac vessels)
- Bilateral absent femoral and distal pulses
- Aorto-iliac bruit

d. How severe is the claudication?

Your examiner will almost certainly ask how you would manage your patient. This is influenced by your assessment of the severity of your patient's claudication.

Use the following parameters:

- What is the claudication distance?
- Can your patient walk *through* the pain?
- How is it affecting your patient's lifestyle or work? (How far do they *need* to walk?)
- Has your patient tried conservative measures, eg stopping smoking, losing weight?
- How rapidly is the problem progressing?

Case 2: Rest pain / Critical ischaemia

The patient will usually be male, aged 60 + .
A strong clue that he has rest pain is if his knee is bent or if his leg is hanging over the bed. Both these positions ease the pain.

The following features differentiate rest pain from claudication:
- The pain is distal, mainly in the toes and forefoot
- Skin pallor
- Trophic changes (page 110)
- Ischaemic ulceration at pressure points (pages 32-33)
- Gangrene: usually dry and wrinkled
- Positive Buerger's test

You may be asked why the pain paricularly occurs at rest.
There are three reasons:
- Decreased arterial flow due to decreased assistance of gravity
- Physiological decreased cardiac output at rest
- Reactive dilatation of skin vessels to warmth (in bed)

Case 3: Diabetic foot

As in the above case, your patient may have ulcers at pressure points and gangrenous toes. Remember that the pathology is multifactorial:
- Arterial occlusive disease
- Microscopic angiopathy
- Peripheral neuropathy (sensory, motor, autonomic)
- Infection

The following features distinguish the diabetic foot from the critically ischaemic foot:
- The patient is younger
- The foot is red and warm
- Gangrene is usually accompanied by infection: there may be deep collections of pus
- The pulses may be present

Case 4: Aortic aneurysm

This is a common short and long case in surgical finals.

As always, look carefully. You may see a pulsating mass in the umbilical region.

An aortic aneurysm has an *expansile* pulsatility as opposed to a *transmitted* pulsatility. To distinguish between these, place the fingers of your two hands on either side of the mass and look to see if they are actually being pushed apart.

Measure the horizontal distance between your fingers: remember that, especially in thin females, the abdominal aorta is easily palpable.

Can your hand get above it? If so, it is infrarenal (most common).

Is the aneurysm tender? This suggests it may be about to rupture (a very unlikely examination situation!)

Auscultate over the swelling: a loud bruit (in the absence of a similar bruit in the heart) supports the diagnosis.

Check the femoral, popliteal and foot pulses. These are usually present, as patients presenting with aneurysms rarely have peripheral vascular disease. However, emboli from the aneurysm may cause distal occlusion.

Case 5: Amputation

Peripheral vascular disease is by far the commonest cause of amputation in the elderly. You may meet such a patient in the long case.

Take a detailed history of the immediate events leading up to the amputation but do not get bogged down in the probably lengthy history of previous operations such as bypasses and sympathectomies.

Your history should be geared largely towards the sociological implications of the amputation. Ask about mobility: can the patient climb stairs? Is he/she likely to be confined to a wheelchair existence? Assess the patient's ability to wash, dress and self care in other ways. Ask also about occupational therapy, home help, aids and appliances.

Determine whether the amputation is below knee/through knee/above knee and look carefully at the wound site. Is it infected? Are there contractures of the hip and knee joints?

POPULAR VIVA QUESTIONS

— Why does critical ischaemia lead to pain at rest?

— What is the cause of a bruit?

— What factors would influence your management of a patient with claudication?

— What are the causes of diabetic foot disease?

— What causes of intermittent claudication would you consider in a young patient?

— What are the causes of an acutely ischaemic limb?

— What are the symptoms and signs of an acutely ischaemic limb?

— What is the *brachio-radial* pressure index? Why measure it?

— What anatomical features on the arteriogram determine the severity of ischaemia in an atherosclerotic limb?

— What are the risk factors for peripheral vascular disease?

THE HISTORY

Include the following questions:

Presenting complaint
— What is your main problem? (The patient may be bothered by the appearance, aches and pains or something else.)

— Are you on your feet all day? Do your legs ache more towards the end of the day?

— How long have you had the problem? Have you seen anyone about it previously? Was it treated then?

Predisposing causes
— Does anyone else in your family have varicose veins?

— Have you ever been pregnant? Did you have any problems with your legs then? Did one leg swell up?

— Have you had any major injuries or operations? Did you have any problems with your legs then? Did one leg swell up?

In your systemic enquiry, ask about abdominal and gynaecological symptoms, particularly,

— Have your noticed any swelling of your abdomen?

— Have your clothes become tighter lately?

THE EXAMINATION

Venous insufficiency is a common short case. Practise the Tourniquct test. It may look easy on paper but the only way it doesn't end up an embarrassing fiasco in front of your examiners is for it to be a well-worn routine. Be absolutely clear about its significance. You may think you understand it but, with exam nerves, explaining it is another matter.

"Examine this patient's varicose veins"

ACTION	NOTE
– Introduce yourself	
– Ask permission to examine the patient	
– Expose both legs with the patient standing up	
LOOK	
– Compare shape of legs	*?beer-bottle leg*
– Observe: • anteriorly • posteriorly	*?distribution of varicose veins*
– Observe skin changes in 'gaitor area' (lower third of leg, especially above medial malleolus)	*?venous stars* *?eczema* *?pigmentation* *?ulcers*
FEEL	
– Run the back of your hand down both legs	*?warm over varicose veins*
– Palpate along the medial side of the lower leg Ask if it is tender	*?tenderness* (occurs at sites of perforators)
– Feel around the ankle	*?dermatoliposclerosis* *?pitting oedema*

– Feel the saphenofemoral junction (4cm below and lateral to pubic tubercle) Ask patient to cough

?saphena varix

?cough impulse (indicates saphenofemoral incompetence)

– Feel the sapheno-popliteal junction (popliteal fossa) Ask patient to cough

?cough impulse (indicates saphenopoplital incompetence)

ASSESS FURTHER

a. Tap Test

– Place the fingers of one hand at the lower limit of a long varicose vein Tap above with your other hand

? percussion impulse: (indicates incompetence of *superficial* veins)

b. Tourniquet Test

– Ask patient to lie down flat
– Elevate one leg until the superficial veins are emptied Place a rubber tourniquet tightly around the upper thigh (If patient is unable to hold up leg, ask the examiner to hold it up)

– Ask patient to stand up
Watch *below* the
tourniquet

*?filling of superficial veins
below tourniquet* (indicates
incompetent perforators *below*
tourniquet)

– Keep repeating the
procedure, moving the
tourniqnet progressively
down the leg
Position the tourniquet
in between the sites of
the perforator veins
(see page 127)
Repeat until the veins
below the tourniquet
stay collapsed

Defines the segment of leg
containing incompetent
perforators

c. Trendelenburg Test

– Ask patient to lie flat

Only perform this test if the
tourniquet test is positive
at upper third of thigh

– Elevate the leg until
the superficial veins
are emptied

Place two fingers at the
saphenofemoral junction

– Ask patient to stand up,
keeping your fingers
firmly in place
Watch leg

*?no filling of superficial
veins below fingers*
(indicates saphenofemoral
incompetence)

d. <u>Perthes Test</u>

– Place a tourniquet
  around leg so that the
  veins below tourniquet
  are empty

– Ask patient to stand up   *?filling of superficial veins*
  and down on tip-toe ten   *on exercise* (indicates deep
  times   venous occlusion)
  Watch leg

e. <u>Listen</u>

– Auscultate over sites of   *?bruit* (indicates AV
  marked venous clusters   malformation - rare)

  SAY

  "I would like to:
    • examine the abdomen   *?abdominal or pelvic mass*
    • do a rectal   (may cause inferior vena caval
      examination   obstruction)
    • do a pelvic
      examination (in
      females)
    • examine the external
      genitalia (in males)"

  **COMPLETE THE
  EXAMINATION**

– Lie the patient down

– Cover the legs

– Turn to your examiner
  and present your findings

TYPICAL CASES

Although a patient with an acute deep vein thrombosis is unlikely to come up in an examination, you should know about the presentation and differential diagnosis of this common emergency.

Be absolutely clear as to what is meant by the terms 'varicose veins' and 'venous insufficiency'. Your patient may have one or both of these conditions.

Case 1:   Varicose veins

Your patient will usually have primary varicose veins, ie no known underlying cause. There may be a positive family history. However, always seek a secondary cause (see history and examination above).

You may be asked to define varicose veins: these are "dilated, tortuous, superficial veins".

A knowledge of the anatomy will help in your description of the distribution of the varicosities. Note that the muscular wall usually prevents dilatation of the *main* leg veins: varicosities occur in the *tributaries*.

a.   The long saphenous vein:

- Arises from the dorsal venous arch
- Runs anterior to the medial malleolus
- Runs behind the medial aspect of the knee
- Runs up the leg superficial to deep fascia
- Pierces cribriform fascia at the saphenous opening
- Empties into the femoral vein

b.   The short saphenous vein:

- Arises from the dorsal venous arch
- Runs behind the lateral malleolus
- Runs up the midline of the calf superficial to deep fascia
- Pierces deep fascia over the popliteal fossa
- Empties into the popliteal vein

c. <u>The perforator veins</u>

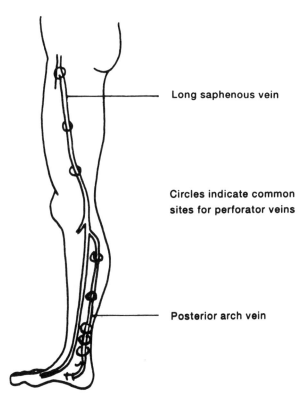

Long saphenous vein

Circles indicate common
sites for perforator veins

Posterior arch vein

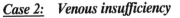

Case 2: *Venous insufficiency*

This describes the following dermatological trial:

- Eczema (a low-grade cellulitis)
- Pigmentation (haemosiderin deposition)
- Venous ulcers (see page 31)

Your examiner will want to know if you have a clear understanding of the difference between *superficial* and *deep* venous insufficiency.

	SUPERFICIAL VENOUS INSUFFICIENCY	DEEP VENOUS INSUFFICIENCY
Aetiology	Primary varicose veins (unknown cause)	A late complication of deep vein thrombosis
Pathogenesis	Incompetent *perforator* veins: causes blood flow from *deep* to *superficial* system	Incompetent *deep* veins: leads to *raised pressure* in deep system. This causes blood flow from *deep* to *superficial* system (NB associated incompetent perforators *may* lead to *secondary* varicose veins)
Skin changes	Mild	Severe: 'beer-bottle leg' due to: • brawny oedema • dermatoliposclerosis (subcutaneous fat replaced by collagen)
Prognosis	Better response to surgery	Worse response to surgery

Case 3: AV malformations

Although AV malformations are rare, they are life-long problems often with good physical signs and they may therefore turn up as short cases.

Consider this diagnosis if you come across an easily compressible, superficial mass of vessels.

The malformation may be *congenital* or *acquired*. In a *congenital* AV malformation, your patient will tell you that the symptoms have been present from birth or childhood. There will often be gigantism of the affected limb. In *acquired* AV fistulae, there is a history of trauma. This may be surgically induced, as in the case of a fistula for haemodialysis.

Look for the following features:
- Signs of venous insufficiency
- Pulsatility
- Hum: always *listen* over large, unusually sited collections of varicosities

POPULAR VIVA QUESTIONS

— Describe the aetiology of varicose veins.

— What do you understand by the term venous insufficiency?

— What are the indications for operating on a person with varicose veins?

— How would an acute deep venous thrombosis present?

— What are the complications of a deep venous thrombosis?

— What are the causes of deep venous thrombosis?

THE HISTORY

Pain

Ask the usual questions about pain (see page 19). Be clear as to where your patient's pain is felt *maximally* and where it *radiates*. Ask specifically if there is any *knee* pain.

When enquiring into exacerbating factors, ask about actions that load the joint, eg putting on socks, sitting in a low chair, rising from a sitting position and walking.

Stiffness

Ask if this is worse in the morning, on movement or after staying in one position.

Walking

— Ask how far the patient can walk.
— Has he/she noticed a limp or change in leg length?
— Ask in detail about aids and applicances: does the patient need a walking stick or a Zimmer frame?

In a long case, you must take a detailed social history. Find out how the problem affects the patient's life-style and whether it is deteriorating. Ask about the involvement of other joints: many patients with osteoarthritis or rheumatoid arthritis of the hip will have had other joint replacements.

THE EXAMINATION

The examination of the hip and knee is where most candidates let themselves down. You will probably not have had nearly as much practice as, say, examining an abdomen. Practise on each other: it is very easy for the examiner to see if you have done it before.

Most of the patients in short cases will have osteoarthritis and will be fairly fragile. If they are supine when you are introduced, it is probably simpler to start examining in this position. However, never forget to stand the patient up to perform the Trendelenburg test and to watch the gait.

In a long case, it is essential to examine the peripheral vascular system and to look for signs of infection in the leg. Both ischaemia and infection could potentially compromise a total hip replacement.

"Examine this patient's hip"

ACTION	NOTE
– Introduce yourself	
– Ask permission to examine the patient	
– Expose both legs with the patient supine	
– Check that the ASISs are at the same level	
LOOK	
– Roll the patient to one side to observe the buttock and posterior thigh	skin: *?scars* *?sinuses* soft tissues: *?swelling* (the hip joint is deep and swelling is not usually seen) muscle: *?gluteal wasting*
– Look at the ankles	bony alignment: *?obvious difference in leg length*

– Look at the position of the patella and foot on each side

?external rotation

– Look at the angle between the thigh and bed

?fixed flexion deformity

MEASURE

If there is a fixed deformity, place unaffected leg in the same position as the affected leg

– Measure from the ASIS to the medial malleolus

?true leg lengths

– Measure from the xiphisternum to the medial malleolus

?apparent leg lengths
see page 140

– If there is any disparity in true leg length, ask the patient to bend the knees, keeping the ankles together
Compare the position of the two knees

?shortening below knee
(tibial shortening)

?shortening above knee
(femoral shortening)

– If shortening is above the knee, put your thumbs on ASISs and feel down with your fingers until you reach the top of the greater trochanters

?Is there a difference in the distance between ASIS and greater trochanter
(suggests shortening is in the hip joint itself)

FEEL

- Ask if there is any tenderness
- Palpate over greater trochanter

  ?tenderness

  T.
  Bone contour
  Stiffness
  Swelling

- Palpate over anterior joint line (just lateral to femoral pulse)

  Tenderness
  Heat and swelling is only felt if patient is very thin

MOVE

a. Thomas' Test and Flexion

see page 141

- Place your left hand in the hollow of the lumbar spine

- Flex the hip and knee of the unaffected side until the lumbar spine straightens

  ?range of flexion of
  unaffected side
  (normally 130°)

- Look to see if hip of the affected side lifts up from the bed

  ?fixed flexion deformity of
  affected hip

- Flex the hip and knee of the affected side

  ?range of flexion of affected
  hip

b. Abduction and Adduction

- Rest your left forearm between the ASISs, keeping one hand on the pelvis

  This stabilises the pelvis

– Hold the ankle with the
other hand

First abduct and then
adduct leg until the
pelvis starts to move

?range of abduction
(normally 45°)

?range of adduction
(normally 30°)

c. Rotation

– Go to the end of the bed
Grasp the ankles and
rotate each leg
internally and
externally
Watch the patellae

Rotation may also be tested
with the hip and knee flexed
to 90°

*?range of internal and
external rotation*
(normally both 45°)

d. Abnormal movement

– Alternately push and
pull the leg along its
long axis

?telescoping (a sign of
marked instability)

STAND

– Look again: • anteriorly

?rotational deformity

• laterally

?pelvic tilt
?increased lumbar lordosis

• posteriorly

?scoliosis
?gluteal wasting

a. Trendelenburg Test

- Sit on a chair, facing
  the patient

- Place one hand on each   The patient may rest his/her
  side of the patient's   hands on your shoulders to
  pelvis   maintain balance

- Ask patient to stand on
  one leg
  Feel if the hip on the   *?hip rises on opposite side*
  opposite side rises or   (negative test - normal)
  falls
                                ?hip falls on opposite side
                                (positive test - abnormal:
                                see page 139)

- Repeat on the opposite
  side

b. Gait

- Ask patient to walk away   *?Trendelenburg gait*
  from you and then   *?antalgic gait*
  towards you   *?supports, eg stick, frame*
  Watch carefully

**COMPLETE THE
EXAMINATION**

- Make sure patient is
  comfortable

- Turn to the examiner

- Present your findings

TYPICAL CASES

Case 1: Hip pain

If you meet a patient with a hip disorder in the long case, he/she will almost certainly complain of pain.

You should know the characteristics of hip pain: this is usually felt maximally in the anterior groin. However, it is poorly-defined and radiates variably to the following areas:

- Anterior thigh
- Lateral thigh
- Buttock
- Anterior knee
- Anterior lower leg

Remember that a patient with a primary hip disorder may present with isolated *knee* pain. This is because both the hip and knee contribute fibres to the obturator and femoral nerves.

Use the following table to differentiate hip pain from other local or distant causes:

	SITE OF MAXIMUM PAIN	RADIATION	EXACERBATING FACTORS
Hip pain	Anterior groin	Wide and variable (see above)	See history above
Trochanteric bursitis	Greater trochanter	Lateral thigh	Lying on affected side
Meralgia paraesthetica (entrapment of lateral cutaneous nerve of thigh)	Anterolateral thigh	None	• Pregnancy • Tight corsets • Jeans
Sacroiliac pain	Deep in buttock	Posterior thigh	Standing on one leg (affected side)
Nerve root pain due to prolapsed disc (L1/L2)	• Groin • Back	None	Straining/ coughing
Ischaemic pain due to aorto-iliac disease (see page 117)	• Calf • Thigh • Buttock	None	Walking

Case 2: *Abnormal gait*

You may be asked to describe the gait of a patient with hip pathology. The two main types are the *Antalgic* gait and the *Trendelenburg* gait *(waddling gait if bilateral).* You should know how they differ:

	ANTALGIC GAIT	**TRENDELENBURG GAIT**
Cause	Painful hip	Inefficient hip abduction
Weight-bearing/ stance phase	Shortened	Pelvis droops on opposite side
Direction to which body leans whilst weight-bearing	Towards affected side	Towards unaffected side

You may be asked to describe the mechanism of the Trendelenburg gait. This is probably best understood by considering the Trendelenburg test:

Normally, when standing on one leg, the abductors on the weight-bearing side contract so that the pelvis rises on the *opposite* side. A positive Trendelenburg test occurs when there is any *inefficiency of hip abduction*: the pelvis droops towards the unsupported side.

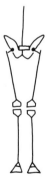

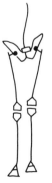

Negative
Trendelenburg test
(normal)

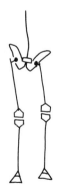

Positive
Trendelenburg test
(abnormal)

Inefficiency of hip abduction occurs as a result of the following:

a. Disturbance in the pivotal mechanism

    (i)   *dislocation* or *subluxation* of the hip
    (ii) *shortening of the femoral neck*

b. Weakness of the hip abductors *(gluteus medius* and *minimus)*

    (i)   *myopathy* (usually *bilateral*)
    (ii) *neuropathy* (L5 root lesion, usually unilateral)

Case 3: Arthritis of the hip

A patient with primary osteoarthritis of the hip is a very common short or long case. You could also be given a patient with rheumatoid arthritis and you should know how to distinguish the two conditions (see pages 151-152).

A patient with osteoarthritis will complain of hip pain (see Case 1). This will initially occur only after activity, but later be present at rest. Look carefully at the gait (see Case 2).

You may be asked the reasons why you measure apparent leg length and perform Thomas' test: arthritis may result in *contractures* which give rise to *deformities*. The most common are fixed *adduction* and *flexion deformities*. Both may be masked by compensatory movements.
The aim of measuring apparent leg length and performing Thomas' test is to *unmask* these contractures:

a. Apparent leg shortening

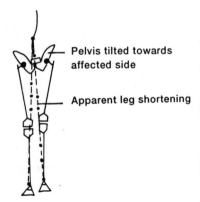

Pelvis tilted towards affected side

Apparent leg shortening

A fixed adduction deformity would tend to cross the legs. Therefore, the pelvis compensates by tilting towards the affected side. This leads to apparent leg shortening.

(True shortening arises from loss of joint space.)

b. Thomas' Test

A fixed flexion deformity can be completely masked by a lumbar lordosis. This is unmasked by performing Thomas' test.

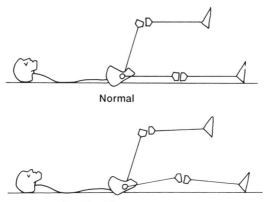

Normal

Positive Thomas Test:
Flexion of normal hip reveals
fixed flexion of the other.

POPULAR VIVA QUESTIONS

— What are the risk factors for congenital dislocation of the hip?

— How do we screen for congenital dislocation of the hip?

— How would you manage a baby presenting with congenital dislocation of the hip?

— What is a slipped upper femoral epiphysis?

— What is Protrusio acetabuli?

— What is Perthes' disease?

— What is the difference between true and apparent leg shortening?

— Describe the radiological appearances of osteoarthritis and rheumatoid arthritis.

— How would you manage a patient with osteoarthritis of the hip?

— What are the operations available for a patient with osteoarthritis of the hip?

— What are the complications of a total hip replacement?

— What are the contra-indications to a total hip replacement?

— Describe Garden's classification of fractured neck of femur. What is its significance?

THE HISTORY

If you have a patient with a knee complaint in the long case, bring out the following aspects in your presentation:

Pain
— Ask the usual questions about pain (see page 19).
  Be very clear as to whether the pain is generalised or localised.
— Tell the patient to point with one finger to where the pain is felt maximally.
— Ask if there is pain *above* the knee.
— Ask if it is exacerbated by walking or walking up and down stairs.

Stiffness
Ask if this is worse in the morning, on movement or after staying in one position.

Swelling
If preceded by an injury,
  — Did the swelling occur straight away?
  — Did the swelling occur after a few hours?

Episodes of locking or giving way
Explain to the patient exactly what you mean by these terms.
'Locking' is the sudden inability to extend the knee fully.
'Giving way' describes the feeling of apprehension on weight bearing.

THE EXAMINATION

As with the hip, examination of the knee will probably be relatively unfamiliar: practise on each other.

Don't worry too much about the 'additional assessment', eg the apprehension test and McMurray's test. Most of your examiners are not orthopaedic surgeons and just want to see that you have a basic routine of **LOOK, MEASURE, FEEL, MOVE.**

Never forget to ask to see the patient *walk* at the end of the examination. This will also give you the opportunity of looking at the popliteal fossa for posterior knee swellings.

"Examine this patient's knee"

ACTION	NOTE
– Introduce yourself	
– Ask permission to examine the patient	
– Expose both legs with the patient lying down	
LOOK	
– Compare the two sides	skin: *?erythema* *?scars* swelling: *?pre-patellar* *?infrapatellar*

MEASURE

– Measure the
circumference of each
leg at a fixed point
above the tibial tuberosity

Initial quadriceps wasting
can be detected just medial
to the upper part of the
patella

FEEL

a. Temperature

– Run the back of your
hand over both legs
anteriorly and down each
side

?warm

b. Tests for effusion

(i) *Bulge Test*

Positive with very *little*
fluid present

– Empty the medial
compartment by massaging
up the medial side of
the joint
Retain fluid in the suprapatellar
bursa with medial pressure
from one hand
Stroke down lateral side
of the joint with your
other hand, watching the
medial side

*?appearance of ripple on
flattened medial surface*

(ii) *Patellar tap*

Positive with *large* effusion

– Empty the suprapatellar
bursa: use your left
hand to press downwards
and inwards above the
patella

Keep this hand in position Push the patella sharply back with your right hand	*?tap of patella on femur*

c. <u>Palpation of joint line</u>

The joint line is lower than you think

– Bend the knee to about 50°
– Palpate the *medial* joint line: locate the tibial tuberosity and move your finger medially and proximally
Palpate firmly, anterior to posterior
Ask if/when it hurts

tenderness: *?localised*
　　　　　　?generalised

synovium:　*?thickened*

cartilage:　*?swelling*

– Palpate the *lateral* joint line moving your finger laterally and proximally

– Palpate the popliteal fossa

?swelling

MOVE

a. <u>Flexion and Extension</u>

– Ask patient to bend and then straighten his/her leg
Ask if/when it hurts

range of active movement:
?limited flexion/extension

– Place your hand over the extended knee

– Try to flex and extend the knee joint yourself

range of passive movement:
?limited flexion/extension
?crepitus

– Try to hyperextend the leg by lifting the heel upwards from the bed

?hyperextension

b. <u>Ligament Stability</u>

   (i) *Medial collateral*
      ligament

– Place one hand on the
  lateral side of the *knee*
  and the other on the
  medial side of the *ankle*
  Try to push the ankle   ?*excess movement*
  laterally while pushing   ?*pain*
  the knee medially

   (ii) *Lateral collateral*
      ligament

– Place one hand on the
  medial side of the *knee*
  and the other on the
  lateral side of the *ankle*   ?*excess movement*
  Try to push the ankle   ?*gap sign* (opening up of
  medially while pushing   lateral joint line)
  the knee laterally   ?*pain*

   (iii) *Anterior cruciate ligament*

– Flex the knee to 90°
  Steady foot by sitting
  close (not on it)

– Palpate the hamstrings
  to ensure they are
  relaxed

– Place thumbs of both
your hands on the tibial
tuberosity
Grasp the lower leg and
pull it towards you

*?tibia displaced anteriorly
on femur* (positive anterior
drawer sign)
There may be a false-positive
anterior drawer sign if the
posterior cruciate ligament is ruptured

(iv) *Posterior cruciate
ligament*

– Repeat above test but
push the tibia *away* from
you

*?tibia displaced posteriorly
on femur* (positive posterior
drawer sign)

ASSESS FURTHER

a. The Apprehension Test

– Hold the patella
laterally with the knee
extended
Bend the knee slowly

Only perform this test if you
suspect patella instability

– Watch patient's face

*?resistance to further
movement*

b. McMurray's Test

– Flex the knee, holding
the joint steady

Only perform this test if you
suspect a torn meniscus

– Use your other hand to
slowly extend the joint as
you rotate the foot first
medially and then laterally

*?resistance to further
movement*
?pain
?click

STAND

– Ask patient to stand up

– Look from:
  • in front
  • the side
  • the back

– Ask patient to walk away
  from you and then
  towards you

**COMPLETE THE
EXAMINATION**

– Make sure patient is
  comfortable

– Turn to the examiner

– Present your findings

Genu valgum and varum are
best seen in standing
position

?genu valgum/varum
?genu recurvatum
?swelling in popliteal fossa

Gait: *?short-stepping*
             ?limp

TYPICAL CASES

As with the hip, pain is the most common presenting symptom. It may be associated with stiffness and mechanical problems.

I. KNEE PAIN

First ask yourself if the pain is due to knee pathology or if it is referred.

	KNEE PATHOLOGY	REFERRED PAIN
Localised?	Yes	No
Any pain above knee?	No	Yes
Exacerbated by walking?	Yes	No

Case 1: *Anterior knee pain*
Patellofemoral abnormalities cause anterior knee pain. This is characteristically exacerbated by the following:
   • Going up and down stairs
   • Sitting for a long time with the knee flexed

You may be asked the causes:

(i)   *Congenital* eg bipartite patella

(ii) *Injuries*

(iii) *Stress*
   • Growth spurt (esp. adolescent females)
   • Chondromalacia patellae (esp. adolescent males)
   • Obesity
   • Synovial shelf syndrome

(iv) *Bone osteochondritis*
  • Osgood-Schlatter's / Sliding Larson's disease
  • Osteochondritis dissecans

(v) *Bursae and diverticulae*
  • Bursitis
  • Popliteal cyst/Baker's cysts

(vi) *Joint pathology*
  • Rheumatoid arthritis
  • Osteoarthritis
  • Tuberculosis

Case 2: *Arthritides*

Compare and contrast the symptoms and signs of rheumatoid arthritis and osteoarthritis:

	OSTEOARTHRITIS	RHEUMATOID ARTHRITIS
Pain	+ +	+ +
Stiffness	+	+ +
Palpable synovium	–	+ +
Deformity	Genu varum	Genu valgum
Effusion	+	+ +
Limitation of movement	+ +	+ +
Crepitus	+ +	+ +
Joint instability	–	+

Ask specifically about the *pattern* of stiffness: this may tell you about the joint pathology:

	OSTEOARTHRITIS	RHEUMATOID ARTHRITIS
Morning stiffness	Sometimes	Very common
Time for morning stiffness to diminish	10 - 20mins (approx)	30 mins - 1 hour (approx)
Stiffness after staying in one position	+ +	+

If you are asked to examine the knee in a short case, always glance at the hands. This will give you a clue if your patient has rheumatoid arthritis.

Remember: the knee may be the only joint involved in osteoarthritis whereas in rheumatoid arthritis, it is usually involved as part of a generalised syndrome.

Look carefully for scars of previous operations: your patient may have had a joint replacement.

Case 3: Mechanical problems

You would be extremely unlikely to have a patient with an acute injury in the examination. However, your patient could be a young man complaining of recurrent episodes of pain and locking following a meniscal tear.

Other causes of locking are *plica syndrome* (trapping of a synovial fold) and *loose bodies ('joint mice')*.

Know the causes of joint mice:
- Osteochondritis dissecans
- Synovial chondromalacia
- Osteochondral fracture
- Localised separation of articular cartilage

A knee 'gives way' in patellofemoral disease and when there is any weakness of the quadriceps, especially vastus medialis.

Case 4: *Knee deformities*

You should know the causes of the two most common deformities, **genu valgum** and **genu varum**:

	GENU VARUM (BOW LEGS)	GENU VALGUM (KNOCK KNEES)
1. Physiological	Babies	Toddlers aged 3-4 (permissable to have 10cm between ankles)
2. Arthritides	Osteoarthritis - cartilage loss in medial compartment	Rheumatoid arthritis
3. Metabolic	Vit C, D deficiency	Vit C, D deficiency
4. Growth disorders	• Paget's disease • Epiphyseal injury • Dysplasias, eg Blount's disease	• Epiphyseal injury • Dysplasias

II. KNEE SWELLINGS

Most lumps in and around the knee are due to bursitis or diverticulae. Know the differential diagnosis:

(i)   *Anterior* (rare)
  • Pre-patellar bursa
    (Housemaid's knee)
  • Infrapatellar bursa
    (Clergyman's knee)
  • Osgood-Schlatter's disease

(ii) *Lateral/Medial* (rare)
  • Cyst of lateral meniscus
  • Cyst of medial meniscus
  • Exostosis

(iii) *Posterior*
  • Semimembranous bursa
  • Baker's cyst
  • Popliteal aneurysm

You should be able to recognise a bursa by the following features:

  • Not tender (unless infected)
  • Smooth surface
  • Fluctuant
  • Transilluminable
  • May be attached to skin
  • Immobile

Case 5: Anterior knee swellings

(i) *Pre-patellar bursitis: housemaid's knee*
Here the swelling is *over* the patella.
Ask the patient his/her occupation: it is common in carpet layers, tilers and roofers, but not so common in housewives!

(ii) *Infrapatellar bursitis: clergyman's knee*
Here the swelling is *distal* to the patella.

(iii) *Osgood-Schlatter's disease*
Suspect this condition in an adolescent who complains of pain after physical activity: look for a lump over the tibial tuberosity. On palpation, it is usually tender.

Case 6: Posterior knee swellings

(i) *Semimembranous bursitis*
The swelling is behind the knee in the medial part of the popliteal fossa, above the joint line.

(ii) *Baker's cyst/Popliteal cyst*
This is a synovial diverticulum extending into the popliteal fossa through a deficit in the posterior capsule.
The swelling is behind the knee, below the joint line.

You may be asked to distinguish the terms 'popliteal cyst' and 'Baker's cyst':

Popliteal Cyst:
 • No underlying pathology
 • Seen in young adults/children

Baker's cyst:
 • Pathology of rest of knee, eg rheumatoid arthritis, osteoarthritis, gout, tuberculosis
 • Often exacerbates pre-existing symptoms, eg further interference with knee flexion

(iii) *Popliteal aneurysm*

This is easily detected because of its *expansile* pulsation.

— Always palpate the other leg (it may be bilateral).
— Examine the peripheral pulses.
— Palpate the abdomen for an associated aortic aneurysm.

POPULAR VIVA QUESTIONS

— What is the normal angle of the femur on the tibia?

— What are the causes of genu varum?

— What are the causes of genu valgum?

— What is the cause of Osgood-Schlatter's disease?

— What is osteochondritis dissecans?

— What are the causes of anterior knee pain?

— What do we mean by 'a locked knee'? When does this occur?

— What radiological features would you see in osteoarthritis?

— What radiological features would you see in rheumatoid arthritis?

— Where is the most common site for a meniscus to tear? How would such an injury present?

15: THE HAND AND FOOT

THE HISTORY

Hand and foot problems usually come up as short cases.

You may be told to ask the patient a few questions: first ask about the patient's main complaint. Then go through the usual questions about pain and swelling (page 19).

Ask specifically about loss of function:
— Can you hold a cup easily?
— Can you turn a doorknob?
— Do you have difficulty dressing yourself, eg doing up buttons?
— Do you have difficulty washing yourself?

THE EXAMINATION

The instruction will usually be to "examine this person's hands". Seek clues as to the underlying cause right from the beginning.
Look at the following:

- Elbows: *?rheumatoid nodules*
- Nails and skin: *?nail pitting ?psoriasis*
- Ears: *?gouty tophi*

"Examine this patient's hand(s)"

ACTION	NOTE
— Introduce yourself	
— Ask permission to examine the patient	
— Place a pillow on the patient's lap and tell the patient to rest *both* hands on it	

LOOK

Observe:

• dorsal surface	skin: *?thin / bruised* nails: *?clubbing / pitting* muscle: *?wasting of dorsal interossei* joints: *?swelling* (Heberden's or Bouchard's nodes) bony deformities: *?rheumatoid arthritis* (page 170)
• palmar surface	skin: *?erythema* *?Dupytren's contracture* muscles: *?wasting of thenar/hypothenar eminence and ventral interossei*
• from the side (patient's hands outstretched)	*?finger drop*
• knuckles (patient's fists clenched)	*?swelling of MCP joints*
• hands in praying position and back to back	Examine bulk of thenar and hypothenar eminences: *?same on both sides*

FEEL

– Ask if hands are painful

– Run the back of your hand
over patient's forearm
and fingers
Compare the temperature   *?warm*
of both sides

– Squeeze gently over:
  • MCP joints 2-5   *?areas of maximum tenderness*
  • IP joints 2-5   *?soft tissue swelling*
                                   ?bony swelling

– Palpate over:
  • thumb joints   *?areas of maximum tenderness*
  • radiocarpal joint   *?soft tissue swelling*
  • inferior radioulnar   *?bony swelling*
    joint

MOVE

– Place your thumb on   *?limited range of movement*
patient's palm and move   *?crepitus from flexor tendon*
each MCP and IP joint in
turn

TEST POWER

- Ask patient to grip two
of your fingers as hard
as possible

?strength of power grip

- Ask patient to oppose
thumb to index finger as
hard as possible
Hook your index finger
under point of contact
Try to pull it through

?strength of precision grip

- Test thumb abduction:
"Point your thumb up
towards your nose. Now
keep it there and don't
let me push it down"

*?strength of abductor
pollicis longus*
(median nerve)

- Test finger adduction:
"Spread your fingers
wide apart. Don't let
me push them together"

?strength of interossei
(ulnar nerve)

TEST SENSATION

- Compare sensation on
each side with a
pinprick over:
  • index finger
  • little finger
  • lateral aspect of
    thumb base

• median nerve
• ulnar nerve
• radial nerve

ASSESS FUNCTION

– Ask patient to undo a button

– Ask patient to write his/her name

ASSESS FURTHER

Only perform the following tests if appropriate

If you suspect carpal tunnel syndrome,

a. Tinel's Sign

– Percuss over the distal skin crease of wrist

?pain/tingling felt over lateral palm

b. Phalen's Test

– Hold the patient's wrist maximally flexed for one minute

?pain/tingling felt over lateral palm

If you suspect ulnar nerve lesion,

c. Froment's Sign

– Ask patient to grasp a piece of paper between the thumb and index finger (using both hands) Try to pull paper away

?flexing of terminal phalanx as you pull away

If patient cannot flex an IP joint,

- Hold middle phalanx still
  Flex distal phalanx
  Hold all fingers down
  except one to be tested
  Tell patient to flex
  that finger

  ?flexion present (indicates flexor digitorum superficialis intact)

If you suspect de Quervain's tenosynovitis,

d. Finkelstein's Test

- Tell patient to grasp
  his thumb in his palm
  Now deviate the fist
  towards the ulnar side

  ?pain (indicates de Quervain's tenosynovitis)

If you are asked to examine a patient's foot, follow the usual routine of 'LOOK, FEEL, MOVE', examining each joint in turn as outlined on page 181. There will usually be an obvious abnormality which you should describe systematically before giving your diagnosis.

TYPICAL CASES

I. THE HAND

Case 1: *Contracted hand*

You may be shown a contracted hand. Your differential diagnosis will include an ulnar nerve palsy (page 166) and Klumpke's palsy (page 167) which both result in a clawed hand. A contracted hand may result from the following conditions:

	CAUSE	JOINTS AFFECTED
Dupuytren's Contracture	• Alcohol/cirrhosis • Phenytoin • Diabetes mellitus	*Flexion* of MCP and PIP joints (affects ring and little fingers)
Volkmann's Contracture	Trauma at/below elbow leads to ischaemia of forearm muscles	*Flexion* of MCP and IP joints. Can be straightened only when wrist is flexed
Shortening of intrinsic hand muscles	• Spasticity • Scarring due to trauma/infection	*Flexion* of MCP joints *Extension* of IP joints *Adduction* of thumb

The most *common* cause of a contracted hand is **Dupuytren's Contracture:**

— Feel for the hard, subcutaneous nodules on the palmer surface.
— Look at the knuckles which may also be thickened (Garrod's pads).
— Look at the other hand.
— Ask to examine the soles of the feet: similar nodules may be felt.

If permitted, ask the following questions to determine the cause:

— Do you drink alcohol? How much per day?
— Do you have diabetes?
— Do you suffer from epilepsy? Are you on Phenytoin?

Case 2: Median nerve lesion

This is usually carpal tunnel syndrome.
You may be asked the associations. Classify your answer:

- Endocrine causes: (acromegaly, myxoedema)
- Connective tissue diseases: (rheumatoid arthritis)
- Fluid retention: (congestive cardiac failure, pregnancy)
- Trauma

Remember the signs:

(i) *Sensory loss*: over lateral $3^1/_2$ digits:
Note that the palm may be spared as the palmar branch of median nerve passes superficial to the flexor retinaculum.

(ii) *Motor loss and wasting*: affects **LOAF**:

> **L**umbricals (lateral two)
> **O**pponens pollicis
> **A**bductor pollicis brevis (easiest to detect)
> **F**lexor pollicis brevis

(iii) *Positive Tinel's sign and Phalen's Test* (see examination scheme, page 163)

Case 3: Ulnar nerve palsy

This is usually due to trauma at the elbow: *look* for scars here.
It may occasionally arise from repeated trauma to the heel of the hand, in which case there is no sensory loss.

Revise the signs:

(i) *Position*: claw hand
(ii) *Sensory loss*: over little and ring fingers
(iii) *Motor loss and wasting*: affects the interossei; most noticeable dorsally. There is weakened finger abduction and adduction.
(iv) *Positive Froment's sign* (see page 163)

Case 4: Radial nerve palsy

The commonest cause is when the patient falls asleep with his/her arm hanging over the edge of the chair ('Saturday Night Palsy'). Remember that the radial nerve lies in the spiral groove and can therefore also be damaged by fractures of the shaft of the humerus.

The main signs are wrist drop and wasting of the posterior forearm muscles. There is very little sensory loss: only over the anatomical snuffbox.

Case 5: Erb's palsy (C5 C6 roots)

The most common causes are birth trauma and injury. The signs are as follows:

(i)   *Position:* arm internally rotated with the forearm pronated and the palm facing backwards (the waiter's tip sign).

(ii) *Sensory loss:* over deltoid.

(iii) *Muscle weakness and wasting:* affects deltoid, most of shoulder rotator muscles, biceps and brachioradialis.

(iv) *Reflexes:* absent biceps and supinator reflexes.

Case 6: Klumpke's palsy (T1 root)

This may be caused by a cervical rib or apical lung tumour (Pancoast's tumour): remember to check for an associated Horner's syndrome - meiosis, ptosis, enophthalmos and anhydrosis.
The hand is clawed and wasted. There is a sensory loss over the inner aspect of the arm and forearm.

CASE	CAUSE	DIAGRAM
Case 7: ***Dropped finger*** • Usually affects little and ring fingers • Finger can be passively extended but drops down upon release	Extensor tendon rupture (close to ulnar styloid)	
Case 8: ***Mallet finger*** • Terminal IP joint cannot be extended	Division of extensor digitorum longus (at base of distal phalanx)	
Case 9: ***Boutonniere's deformity*** • Flexion of PIP joint • Hyperextension of DIP joint	Rupture of central slip of extensor expansion. Associated with rheumatoid arthritis	

Case 10: **Swan neck deformity** (opposite of Boutonniere's deformity) • Hyperextension of PIP joint • Flexion of DIP joint	Associated with rheumatoid arthritis	
Case 11: **Trigger finger/ Stenosing tenosynovitis** • Patient's finger clicks when it is bent • When patient straightens out hand, affected finger remains bent and then straightens with a click • Feel for a tender nodule over the tendon sheath	Inflammatory thickening of the tendon or its sheath	

Case 12: *Rheumatoid arthritis*

This is a very common short case. You should be able to describe the characteristic deformities:

- Ulnar deviation of the fingers
- Boutonniere's deformity
- Swan neck deformity
- Z-deformity of the thumb
- Subluxation of the MCP joints
- Dorsal subluxation of the ulna at the carpal joint

Also look for the following additional features:

- Swelling of the PIP joints
- Wasting of the small hand muscles
- Atrophic skin and purpura (secondary to steroid therapy)

Palpate the elbows for rheumatoid nodules.

Case 13: *Osteoarthritis*

Note especially,

- Heberden's nodes: bony thickening of DIP joints
- Bouchard's nodes: bony thickening of the PIP joints
- Squaring of thumb: involvement of carpometacarpal joint of thumb

Case 14: *The wasted hand*

This is a common short case.

The two most common causes of generalised hand wasting are old age and rheumatoid arthritis.

However, remember neurological causes:

- – Palpate for a cervical rib.
- – Look for scars around the elbow (ulnar nerve palsy).
- – Test abductor pollicis brevis and the interossei for median and ulnar nerve palsies respectively.

II. DISORDERS OF THE FOOT

The three common foot problems you will see in an examination are hallux valgus, hammer toe and claw toes.

Case 15: Hallux valgus (bunions)
This condition is usually bilateral: always look at the other foot.
Examine for the following features:

- Inflammation: heat and redness over the bunion
- Associated hammer toe
- Corns and collosities over and under the metatarsal heads
- Secondary osteoarthritis of the metatarsophalangeal joint

Case 16: Hammer toe
This usually affects the second toe. It may be bilateral.
There is a fixed flexion deformity of the PIP joint.

Case 17: Claw toes
Claw toes are usually idiopathic. However, you should know the secondary causes:

- Rheumatoid arthritis
- Neurological problems, eg polio, Charcot-Marie-Tooth disease, diabetes

Look for an associated pes cavus (high foot arch).

POPULAR VIVA QUESTIONS

I. THE HAND

— What muscles do the median, ulnar and radial nerves supply in the hand?

— What are the signs of median, ulnar and radial nerve palsies?

— What are the causes of median, ulnar and radial nerve palsies?

— In what position would you fix the hand after injury to avoid stiffness?

— What is de Quervain's tenosynovitis?

— What is a trigger finger?

— What associations of Dupytren's contracture do you know?

II. THE FOOT

— Describe the deformity of club foot.

— Are there any indications for treating flat feet?

— What is hallux valgus? How would you manage it?

— What is the difference between hallux valgus and hallux rigidus?

— What are the causes of pes cavus and claw toes?

16: THE POSTOPERATIVE PATIENT

Surgical wards have a high proportion of postoperative patients who are readily available for examinations. Patients who have recently undergone vascular, gastro-intestinal or transplant surgery may come up as long cases.

In any part of the clinical examination, expect questions on postoperative complications (eg pain, respiratory problems, wounds) and fluid balance. Familiarise yourself with bedside charts which may be used as a basis for discussion.

THE HISTORY

Take a history of both the presenting complaint (ie circumstances that led up to this admission) *and* postoperative events. Screen for common postoperative complications by asking the following questions:

Pain
— Are you in any pain? (Ask specifically about leg pain, chest pain and increasing wound pain.)

Respiratory symptoms:
— Since the operation, have you:
    • been short of breath?
    • had a cough?
    • coughed up blood?

Gastro-intestinal symptoms:
— Have you passed a motion or flatus since the operation?
— Have you noticed any swelling of your abdomen?
— How is your appetite?
— Are you able to eat normally?
— Do you have any nausea or vomiting?

Urinary symptoms

— Did you have a catheter?
— Have you passed urine since the operation?
— Have you had any difficulty passing urine?
— Is there any pain when you pass urine?

Ask also about drugs, including analgesia, antibiotics and heparin prophylaxis.

Take a detailed social history: does the patient live alone? Who will look after him/her after leaving hospital? On which floor does the patient live: are there many stairs to climb / do the lifts work?

THE EXAMINATION

When you examine a postoperative patient, first take a note of the tubes and measuring devices around the bed. Then go on to examine the patient. Finally, never omit to look at observation, fluid and drug charts which will probably be available.

Follow the scheme below:

"Examine this postoperative patient"

ACTION	NOTE
LOOK AROUND THE BED	
• Drips	*?number* *?sites* *?fluid type* *?rate of delivery*
• Lines	*?central venous line* *?arterial line*

• Drains	*?number*
	?site
	bag contents:*?amount*
	?colour
	?blood
	seal: *?sealed unit*
	?underwater seal
• Nasogastric tube	bag contents:*?amount*
	?colour
• Urinary catheter	*?open bag*
	?wash-out attachment
	?volume of urine
	?blood in urine

EXAMINE PATIENT

a. <u>Preliminary assessment</u>

– Form a general impression of the patient	*?ill*
	?in pain
	?evidence of recent weight loss
	?hydration status
– Check the mental state	*?orientated in time/place/person*
– Look at the hands	*?pale skin creases* (clinically anaemic)
– Take the pulse	
– Take the blood pressure	

– Look at the eyes	*?sunken* (dehydration)
– Look at the conjunctivae	*?pale* (clinically anaemic)
– Look at the sclerae	*?jaundice*
– Pinch skin on abdomen	*?lack of skin turgor* (dehydration)

b. <u>Examine the chest</u> (see medical text)

signs of: *?infection*
           ?atelectasis
           ?fluid overload
           ?dehydration

c. <u>Examine the abdomen</u> (page 71)

Ileus may lead to absent bowel sounds after abdominal or retroperitoneal surgery

d. <u>Examine the wound</u>

?site
?type
?stitches/clips
?apposition of edges
?redness
?swelling
?bruising
?copious discharge

e. <u>Examine the legs</u>

?swelling
?tenderness over calf

f. <u>Examine the pressure areas:</u>

  • sacrum
  • heels
  • elbows

?bedsores

LOOK AT THE CHARTS

– temperature chart

        ?pyrexia

– nursing observations

        ?pulse
        ?blood pressure
        ?respiratory rate

– fluid balance

        ?input = output

– drug chart

        ?type of analgesia
        ?drugs for medical problems

COMPLETE THE EXAMINATION

– Make sure your patient
   is comfortable

– Turn to the examiner and
   present your findings

POPULAR VIVA QUESTIONS

— What is the normal daily requirement of water, sodium and potassium?

— How would you determine the amount of fluid to prescribe in the first 24 hours after a laparotomy?

— How would you assess dehydration/overhydration?

— What is the difference between a crystalloid and a colloid?

— What are the complications of blood transfusion?

— Define oliguria.

— How would you manage a patient with oliguria for more than 24 hours postoperatively?

— How would you manage a patient with an increased pulse rate and drop in blood pressure postoperatively?

— Tell me about prophylaxis against deep vein thrombosis.

— What are the possible causes of a pyrexia between 2-10 days post surgery?

— What are some of the alternatives for pain relief post surgery?

— What are some of the predisposing factors for wound infection?

— What are the respiratory complications after major surgery?

— How would you manage a patient with (a) insulin-dependent and (b) non-insulin dependent diabetes pre, peri, and postoperatively?

17: GENERAL APPROACHES

Most of this book is devoted to specific systems or parts of the body. This chapter gives examination schemes which are applicable to more than one system.

Included are approaches to '*a limb*' and '*a joint*'.

I. A LIMB

You may be told to examine a limb, with no clues from the examiner as to which system is abnormal. Always approach the problem by looking systematically and remarking on any abnormalities you see. Then go on to examine the appropriate systems.

The scheme on the following page gives one approach to examining a leg.

"Examine this patient's leg"

	NOTE	
LOOK		see page:
a. <u>Skin</u>	*?varicose veins/signs of venous insufficiency*	126-128
	?trophic changes/ ischaemic ulceration/ gangrene	110
b. <u>Soft tissues</u>	*?swelling of knee*	154
	?quadriceps wasting	145
	?gluteal wasting	132
c. <u>Bony alignment</u>	*?genu varum/valgum*	153
	?disparity in leg length	140
FEEL	- Feel pulses - Check for lymphadenopathy	
MOVE	- Check passive and active movement of each joint - Feel for crepitus	
NEURO-LOGICAL ASSESSMENT	- Test response to light touch (using cotton wool) - Test response to a pin-prick	

II. A JOINT

The most common orthopaedic long and short cases are hips and knees. However, do not panic if you are given a shoulder, an elbow, an ankle or a back to examine. Follow the same routine for all joints:

"Examine this patient's joint"

<u>ACTION</u>	<u>NOTE</u>	
LOOK	skin:	*?erythema*
		?scars
		?sinuses
	soft tissue:	*?swelling*
	muscle:	*?wasting*
	bony alignment:	
		?deformity
FEEL		
– Ask if there is any tenderness		
– Run the back of your hand over joint	temperature: *?warm*	
– Feel any swelling	swelling:	*?fluid*
		?soft tissue
		?bony
- Feel over the joint line	*?tenderness*	

MOVE

– Ask patient to move the joint in each direction in turn

?range of active movement

– Move joint in all directions, feeling for crepitus

?range of passive movement
?crepitus

GENERAL SURGICAL TEXTS

Essential Surgery: Problems, diagnosis and management.
Burkitt H G, 2nd edition, Churchill Livingstone 1995.
A popular textbook of general surgery aimed at clinical medical students. Its main advantages are its very readable style, clear explanations of the pathophysiological basis of surgical problems and illustrated synopses of the main stages of common surgical operations.

Lecture Notes in General Surgery.
Ellis H and Calne R, 8th edition, Blackwell Scientific 1992.
In this text, each surgical disease is consistently classified with useful sections on pathology and management. This is especially helpful for knowing how to structure essay questions.

Surgical Diagnosis and Management: A Guide to General Surgical Care.
Dunn D C and Rawlinson J N, 2nd edition, Blackwell Scientific 1991.
This well-structured text strikes a balance between explaining general principles and giving practical details for the day-to-day management of surgical patients (eg. when drains and sutures come out). It will be particularly useful on the wards in the final year and during house jobs.

An Introduction to the Symptoms and Signs of Surgical Disease.
Browse N, 2nd edition, Edward Arnold 1991.
This is a very thorough guide to surgical examination technique and differential diagnosis of common signs. It is very useful for reference but you may find a smaller, more concise guide more practical for carrying about on the wards.

Clinical Examination of the Patient.
Lumley J S P and Bouloux P M G, Butterworth Heinemann 1994.
This pocket reference book, illustrated with 468 colour photographs, serves as a useful guide for formulating and perfecting your clinical examination technique for finals.

Bailey and Love's New Short Practice of Surgery.
Mann C V, Russell R C G, Williams N S, 22nd edition, Chapman and Hall 1995.
A complete reference surgical textbook if you are unsure of a particular point.

Spot Diagnosis in General Surgery.
Ellis H, 2nd edition, Blackwell Scientific 1993.
A collection of colour photographs of patients, pathology specimens and X-rays. Each photograph is accompanied by background information and relevant questions. A useful revision aid for the short cases and viva.

Oxford Handbook of Clinical Surgery.
McLatchie G R, Oxford University Press 1990.
This pocket handbook is useful for carrying about on the wards. It is full of management plans and practical procedures. However there is not much explanation of basic principles and, while structured, the format is not consistent. It should not be mistaken for a basic surgical text.

Pocket Examiner in Surgery.
Northover J and Treasure T, 2nd edition, Churchill Livingstone 1996.
This pocket book is full of questions and answers and is very useful for carrying around on the wards and quizzing each other when bored or waiting for teaching.

ORTHOPAEDIC TEXTS

Concise System of Orthopaedics and Fractures.
Apley A G and Solomon L, 2nd edition, Butterworth Heinemann 1991.
A popular basic orthopaedics book, full of useful sketches, photographs and X-rays which bring the text to life. Includes examination schemes for different joints.

Clinical Orthopaedic Examination.
McRae R, 3rd edition, Churchill Livingstone 1990.
A very thorough guide to examining orthopaedic cases. Each step in the examination schemes is clearly illustrated with a line drawing. Reading this textbook is the nearest you will get to being taught at the bedside.

Essentials of Orthopaedic Examination.
Hammer A, 3rd edition, Edward Arnold 1994.
A small, clearly illustrated book which adopts a systematic approach to its examination schemes.

Physical Signs in Orthopaedics.
Klenerman L and Walsh H J, BMJ Publishing Group 1994.
Over 200 black and white photographs with questions and answers. A useful revision aid, particularly for spot diagnoses in the short cases.